The Natural Path To Healing your Cardiovascular System

Luna Parnell

Table of Contents

Introduction

The cardiovascular system, also known as the circulatory system, is responsible for the transportation of blood, nutrients, gases, and waste products throughout the body. This system is essential for maintaining homeostasis and overall bodily function. It consists of three main components: the heart, blood vessels, and blood.

Heart

Structure:

- Location: The heart is located in the thoracic cavity between the lungs, slightly left of the midline.
- Layers: The heart wall consists of three layers:
    - Epicardium: The outer layer, which is also the inner layer of the pericardium (a double-walled sac surrounding the heart).
    - Myocardium: The thick middle layer composed of cardiac muscle cells responsible for the heart's contractile function.

- Endocardium: The inner layer, a smooth lining for the chambers of the heart and the valves.
- Chambers: The heart has four chambers:
    - Right Atrium: Receives deoxygenated blood from the body through the superior and inferior vena cava.
    - Right Ventricle: Pumps deoxygenated blood to the lungs via the pulmonary artery.
    - Left Atrium: Receives oxygenated blood from the lungs via the pulmonary veins.
    - Left Ventricle: Pumps oxygenated blood to the body through the aorta.
- Valves: Four valves ensure unidirectional blood flow:
    - Tricuspid Valve: Between the right atrium and right ventricle.
    - Pulmonary Valve: Between the right ventricle and pulmonary artery.
    - Mitral Valve: Between the left atrium and left ventricle.
    - Aortic Valve: Between the left ventricle and aorta.

Function:

- Pumping Mechanism: The heart pumps blood through two main circuits:
    - Pulmonary Circulation: The right side of the heart pumps deoxygenated blood to the lungs for oxygenation.
    - Systemic Circulation: The left side of the heart pumps oxygenated blood to the rest of the body.
- Electrical Conduction System: The heart's rhythmic contractions are regulated by the electrical conduction system, which includes the sinoatrial (SA) node, atrioventricular (AV) node, bundle of His, and Purkinje fibers.

Blood Vessels

Types of Blood Vessels:

- Arteries: Thick-walled vessels that carry oxygen-rich blood away from the heart to the tissues.
    - Structure: Composed of three layers (tunica intima, tunica media, and tunica externa).

- o   Aorta: The largest artery, originating from the left ventricle.
- Veins: Vessels that return deoxygenated blood back to the heart.
  - o   Structure: Thinner walls compared to arteries, with valves to prevent backflow.
  - o   Superior and Inferior Vena Cava: The largest veins, returning blood to the right atrium.
- Capillaries: Microscopic vessels that connect arteries and veins.
  - o   Function: Facilitate the exchange of oxygen, nutrients, and waste products between blood and tissues.
  - o   Structure: Thin walls composed of a single layer of endothelial cells.

Functions:

- Arteries: Transport oxygenated blood at high pressure.
- Veins: Return deoxygenated blood at low pressure.
- Capillaries: Sites of nutrient and gas exchange.

Blood

Components:

- Red Blood Cells (Erythrocytes):
  - Function: Transport oxygen from the lungs to tissues and carbon dioxide from tissues to the lungs.
  - Structure: Biconcave discs without nuclei, containing hemoglobin.
- White Blood Cells (Leukocytes):
  - Function: Part of the immune system, defending the body against infections.
  - Types: Includes neutrophils, lymphocytes, monocytes, eosinophils, and basophils.
- Platelets (Thrombocytes):
  - Function: Play a key role in blood clotting and wound healing.
  - Structure: Small, cell fragment without a nucleus.
- Plasma:
  - Function: The liquid component of blood, transporting nutrients, hormones, and waste products.
  - Composition: Mostly water, containing proteins (albumin, fibrinogen, globulins),

electrolytes, nutrients, and waste
products.

Functions:

- Transport: Carries oxygen, nutrients, hormones, and waste products.
- Regulation: Maintains body temperature, pH balance, and fluid volume.
- Protection: Contains components of the immune system and clotting factors.

The cardiovascular system is an intricate and essential network responsible for sustaining life by delivering oxygen and nutrients to cells, removing waste products, and supporting immune functions. Understanding its components—the heart, blood vessels, and blood—provides insight into the vital processes that maintain homeostasis and overall health.

The Heart: A Detailed Overview

The heart is a muscular organ that serves as the central pump of the cardiovascular system. It is responsible for circulating blood throughout the body, delivering oxygen and nutrients to tissues, and removing waste products. Let's delve into the anatomy and function of the heart in great detail.

Location:

- The heart is located in the thoracic cavity, slightly left of the midline, between the lungs and behind the sternum. It rests on the diaphragm and is protected by the rib cage.

Size and Shape:

- The heart is approximately the size of a clenched fist and weighs between 250-350 grams (9-12 ounces) in adults. It has a conical shape with the apex pointing downwards and to the left, and the base positioned upwards.

Layers of the Heart Wall:

1. **Epicardium:**
    - The outermost layer of the heart wall.
    - It is a thin, serous membrane that also forms the inner layer of the pericardium.
    - Provides a smooth, frictionless surface for the heart.
2. **Myocardium:**
    - The thick, middle layer composed of cardiac muscle cells (myocytes).
    - Responsible for the contractile force of the heart.
    - Contains intercalated discs, which facilitate rapid and coordinated contraction.
3. **Endocardium:**
    - The innermost layer, a smooth endothelial lining for the chambers and valves.
    - Helps reduce friction as blood flows through the heart.
    - Continuous with the endothelium of the blood vessels.

Chambers and Valves

Chambers: The heart has four chambers:

1. **Right Atrium**:
    - Receives deoxygenated blood from the body through the superior and inferior vena cava.
    - Contains the sinoatrial (SA) node, the primary pacemaker of the heart.
2. **Right Ventricle**:
    - Pumps deoxygenated blood to the lungs through the pulmonary artery for oxygenation.
    - Separated from the right atrium by the tricuspid valve.
3. **Left Atrium**:
    - Receives oxygenated blood from the lungs through the pulmonary veins.
    - Separated from the left ventricle by the mitral valve.
4. **Left Ventricle**:
    - Pumps oxygenated blood to the body through the aorta.
    - Has the thickest myocardium due to the high pressure required to pump blood throughout the body.

Valves: The heart contains four valves that ensure unidirectional blood flow:

1. **Tricuspid Valve**:
   - Located between the right atrium and right ventricle.
   - Has three cusps (flaps) that prevent backflow of blood during ventricular contraction.
2. **Pulmonary Valve**:
   - Located between the right ventricle and pulmonary artery.
   - Prevents backflow of blood into the right ventricle after it is pumped to the lungs.
3. **Mitral Valve (Bicuspid Valve)**:
   - Located between the left atrium and left ventricle.
   - Has two cusps and prevents backflow of blood during ventricular contraction.
4. **Aortic Valve**:
   - Located between the left ventricle and aorta.
   - Prevents backflow of blood into the left ventricle after it is pumped into the systemic circulation.

Blood Flow Through the Heart

1. **Deoxygenated Blood Flow:**
    o   Deoxygenated blood from the body enters the right atrium via the superior and inferior vena cava.
    o   Blood flows through the tricuspid valve into the right ventricle.
    o   During ventricular contraction, blood is pumped through the pulmonary valve into the pulmonary artery and to the lungs for oxygenation.
2. **Oxygenated Blood Flow:**
    o   Oxygenated blood from the lungs enters the left atrium via the pulmonary veins.
    o   Blood flows through the mitral valve into the left ventricle.
    o   During ventricular contraction, blood is pumped through the aortic valve into the aorta and distributed to the body.

Electrical Conduction System

The heart's rhythmic contractions are controlled by an intrinsic electrical conduction system:

1. **Sinoatrial (SA) Node**:
   - Located in the right atrium.
   - Acts as the primary pacemaker, generating electrical impulses that initiate each heartbeat.
2. **Atrioventricular (AV) Node**:
   - Located at the junction of the atria and ventricles.
   - Delays the electrical impulse slightly to allow the atria to complete contraction before the ventricles contract.
3. **Bundle of His (Atrioventricular Bundle)**:
   - Pathway for electrical signals from the AV node to the ventricles.
   - Splits into right and left bundle branches.
4. **Purkinje Fibers**:
   - Network of fibers that spread throughout the ventricles.
   - Conduct electrical impulses rapidly to ensure coordinated ventricular contraction.

Coronary Circulation

The heart has its own blood supply, known as coronary circulation:

1. **Coronary Arteries**:
    - Right and left coronary arteries arise from the base of the aorta.
    - They branch into smaller arteries that supply oxygenated blood to the myocardium.
2. **Coronary Veins**:
    - Collect deoxygenated blood from the myocardium.
    - Converge to form the coronary sinus, which empties into the right atrium.

Cardiac Cycle

The cardiac cycle consists of two main phases:

1. **Systole**:
    - Contraction phase.
    - Ventricles contract, pumping blood into the pulmonary artery and aorta.
2. **Diastole**:
    - Relaxation phase.
    - Ventricles relax, allowing them to fill with blood from the atria.

The heart's function and efficiency are assessed using various parameters such as heart rate,

stroke volume, cardiac output, and ejection
fraction.

The heart is a complex, vital organ with a
sophisticated structure and function. It works
tirelessly to pump blood throughout the body,
maintaining the flow of oxygen and nutrients
essential for life. Understanding the heart's
anatomy and physiology provides a foundation
for appreciating its critical role in health and
disease.

Herbs, Vitamins, Minerals, and Supplements for Heart Health

To support and maintain a healthy heart,
various natural remedies, including herbs,
vitamins, minerals, and supplements, can be
incorporated into your daily regimen. Here are
some key ones:

Herbs

1. **Hawthorn:**
     - Benefits: Improves heart
       function, increases blood flow,

reduces blood pressure, and helps in treating heart failure.

- o Active Compounds: Flavonoids, oligomeric procyanidins.
- o Usage: Often taken as a tea, tincture, or capsule.

2. **Garlic**:
   - o Benefits: Lowers blood pressure, reduces cholesterol levels, and possesses anti-inflammatory properties.
   - o Active Compounds: Allicin, sulfur compounds.
   - o Usage: Consumed fresh, as an extract, or in supplement form.

3. **Motherwort**:
   - o Benefits: Acts as a mild sedative, reduces anxiety, and supports heart function, particularly in cases of palpitations.
   - o Active Compounds: Leonurine, stachydrine.
   - o Usage: Typically taken as a tea or tincture.

4. **Ginkgo Biloba**:
   - o Benefits: Improves blood circulation, especially in peripheral areas, and has antioxidant properties.

- o   Active Compounds: Flavonoids, terpenoids.
- o   Usage: Available in extract or capsule form.

Vitamins

1. **Vitamin D**:
   - o   Benefits: Maintains normal blood pressure, supports heart muscle function, and reduces inflammation.
   - o   Sources: Sunlight exposure, fatty fish, fortified foods.
   - o   Supplementation: Often taken as vitamin D3 supplements.
2. **Vitamin B6 (Pyridoxine) and Vitamin B12 (Cobalamin)**:
   - o   Benefits: Reduce homocysteine levels, lowering the risk of cardiovascular diseases.
   - o   Sources: Meat, fish, dairy products, fortified cereals.
   - o   Supplementation: Available as individual supplements or part of a B-complex vitamin.
3. **Vitamin C**:
   - o   Benefits: Acts as an antioxidant, strengthens blood vessels, and supports collagen production.

- Sources: Citrus fruits, berries, bell peppers, broccoli.
- Supplementation: Commonly taken as ascorbic acid supplements.

Minerals

1. **Magnesium**:
    - Benefits: Maintains normal heart rhythm, relaxes blood vessels, and lowers blood pressure.
    - Sources: Nuts, seeds, whole grains, leafy green vegetables.
    - Supplementation: Available as magnesium citrate, magnesium oxide, and other forms.
2. **Potassium**:
    - Benefits: Regulates blood pressure, fluid balance, and supports proper heart function.
    - Sources: Bananas, oranges, potatoes, spinach.
    - Supplementation: Often included in multivitamins or available as potassium chloride supplements.
3. **Calcium**:
    - Benefits: Essential for muscle contractions, including the heart,

and helps maintain blood pressure.
  - ○ Sources: Dairy products, fortified plant-based milks, leafy greens.
  - ○ Supplementation: Available as calcium carbonate, calcium citrate, and other forms.

Supplements

1. **Omega-3 Fatty Acids**:
   - ○ Benefits: Reduce triglycerides, lower blood pressure, decrease the risk of heart disease, and have anti-inflammatory effects.
   - ○ Sources: Fatty fish (salmon, mackerel), flaxseeds, chia seeds.
   - ○ Supplementation: Commonly taken as fish oil or flaxseed oil supplements.
2. **Coenzyme Q10 (CoQ10)**:
   - ○ Benefits: Supports energy production in heart cells, reduces oxidative stress, and improves heart function.
   - ○ Sources: Meat, fish, nuts, some vegetables.
   - ○ Supplementation: Available as ubiquinone or ubiquinol supplements.

3. **L-Arginine**:
    - Benefits: Improves blood flow by producing nitric oxide, which relaxes blood vessels and lowers blood pressure.
    - Sources: Meat, dairy products, nuts, and seeds.
    - Supplementation: Often taken as an amino acid supplement in powder or capsule form.

Thoracic Cavity

The thoracic cavity is a central compartment of the body's chest region, playing a crucial role in respiratory, cardiovascular, and protective functions. It houses essential organs, blood vessels, and structures that are vital for life. Here's a detailed examination of the thoracic cavity:

Location:

- The thoracic cavity is situated in the upper part of the trunk, bounded superiorly by the thoracic inlet (opening at the base of the neck) and inferiorly by the diaphragm (a muscular partition that separates it from the abdominal cavity).

Boundaries:

- **Anterior Boundary**: The sternum (breastbone) and the costal cartilages of the ribs.
- **Posterior Boundary**: The thoracic vertebrae (part of the spine).
- **Lateral Boundaries**: The ribs and the intercostal muscles (muscles between the ribs).

- **Superior Boundary**: The thoracic inlet, which includes structures such as the trachea, esophagus, and major blood vessels.
- **Inferior Boundary**: The diaphragm, a dome-shaped muscle essential for breathing.

Contents of the Thoracic Cavity

The thoracic cavity is divided into three major compartments:

1. **Pleural Cavities (Two)**:
    - Each pleural cavity surrounds one lung and contains a small amount of pleural fluid, which reduces friction during breathing.
    - **Lungs**: The primary organs of the respiratory system, responsible for gas exchange (oxygen and carbon dioxide).
    - **Pleura**: A double-layered membrane that covers the lungs (visceral pleura) and lines the thoracic cavity (parietal pleura).
2. **Mediastinum**:
    - The central compartment of the thoracic cavity, located between the two pleural cavities.

- Structures within the
  Mediastinum:
  - **Heart**: The muscular organ that pumps blood throughout the body.
  - **Pericardium**: The double-walled sac that encloses the heart, providing protection and reducing friction.
  - **Great Vessels**: Includes the aorta, superior and inferior vena cava, pulmonary arteries, and veins.
  - **Trachea**: The windpipe, which conducts air to and from the lungs.
  - **Esophagus**: The muscular tube that carries food and liquids from the throat to the stomach.
  - **Thymus**: An organ involved in the development of the immune system, particularly during childhood.

- **Lymph Nodes and Vessels**: Part of the lymphatic system, involved in immune responses and fluid balance.
- **Nerves**: Including the phrenic nerves (control the diaphragm) and the vagus nerves (part of the autonomic nervous system).

Functions of the Thoracic Cavity

1. **Respiration**:
   - Houses the lungs and the respiratory passages (trachea, bronchi), facilitating the exchange of oxygen and carbon dioxide.
   - The diaphragm and intercostal muscles play a key role in the mechanical process of breathing.
2. **Cardiovascular Function**:
   - Encloses the heart and major blood vessels, enabling the circulation of blood throughout the body.
3. **Protection**:

- The rib cage provides a sturdy protective barrier for the vital organs (heart and lungs) within the thoracic cavity.
    - The sternum and thoracic vertebrae also contribute to the structural protection.
4. **Support and Conduit**:
    - The thoracic cavity provides pathways for structures passing between the neck and the abdomen, such as the esophagus and major blood vessels.

Herbs, Vitamins, Minerals, and Supplements for Thoracic Health

Supporting the health of the organs and structures within the thoracic cavity can be achieved through a variety of natural remedies, including herbs, vitamins, minerals, and supplements. These can help maintain respiratory health, cardiovascular function, and overall thoracic integrity.

Herbs

1. **Eucalyptus**:
    - **Benefits**: Known for its anti-inflammatory and decongestant properties, it helps clear respiratory passages and supports lung function.
    - **Usage**: Often used in essential oil form for inhalation or in teas and lozenges.
2. **Mullein**:
    - **Benefits**: Soothes the respiratory tract, reduces inflammation, and aids in clearing mucus from the lungs.
    - **Usage**: Typically taken as a tea or tincture.
3. **Hawthorn**:
    - **Benefits**: Supports cardiovascular health by improving heart function, increasing blood flow, and reducing blood pressure.
    - **Usage**: Available as a tea, tincture, or in capsule form.
4. **Thyme**:
    - **Benefits**: Acts as an expectorant, antimicrobial, and

anti-inflammatory agent, helping to support respiratory health.

- **Usage**: Can be used in cooking, as a tea, or in essential oil form.

Vitamins

1. **Vitamin C**:
   - **Benefits**: Acts as an antioxidant, supports immune function, and helps in the maintenance of healthy lung tissue.
   - **Sources**: Citrus fruits, berries, bell peppers, broccoli.
   - **Supplementation**: Commonly taken as ascorbic acid supplements.
2. **Vitamin D**:
   - **Benefits**: Essential for immune health, reduces inflammation, and supports overall respiratory and cardiovascular function.
   - **Sources**: Sunlight exposure, fatty fish, fortified foods.
   - **Supplementation**: Often taken as vitamin D3 supplements.
3. **Vitamin E**:
   - **Benefits**: Protects lung tissues from oxidative damage and supports immune function.

- ○ **Sources**: Nuts, seeds, spinach, and broccoli.
- ○ **Supplementation**: Available in capsule or liquid form.

Minerals

1. **Magnesium**:
   - ○ **Benefits**: Essential for muscle function, including the diaphragm and intercostal muscles involved in breathing, and supports cardiovascular health.
   - ○ **Sources**: Nuts, seeds, whole grains, leafy green vegetables.
   - ○ **Supplementation**: Available as magnesium citrate, magnesium oxide, and other forms.
2. **Zinc**:
   - ○ **Benefits**: Supports immune function, helps in the maintenance of respiratory health, and reduces inflammation.
   - ○ **Sources**: Meat, shellfish, legumes, seeds.
   - ○ **Supplementation**: Often taken as zinc gluconate or zinc citrate supplements.

3. **Potassium**:
    - **Benefits**: Maintains fluid and electrolyte balance, supports normal heart function, and aids in muscle contractions.
    - **Sources**: Bananas, oranges, potatoes, spinach.
    - **Supplementation**: Often included in multivitamins or available as potassium chloride supplements.

Supplements

1. **Omega-3 Fatty Acids**:
    - **Benefits**: Reduce inflammation, support cardiovascular health, and improve lung function.
    - **Sources**: Fatty fish (salmon, mackerel), flaxseeds, chia seeds.
    - **Supplementation**: Commonly taken as fish oil or flaxseed oil supplements.
2. **N-acetylcysteine (NAC)**:
    - **Benefits**: Acts as an antioxidant, helps clear mucus, and supports lung health.
    - **Sources**: Not commonly found in foods; primarily taken as a supplement.

- o **Supplementation**: Available in capsule or powder form.

3. **Coenzyme Q10 (CoQ10)**:
   - o **Benefits**: Supports heart health by aiding in energy production and reducing oxidative stress.
   - o **Sources**: Meat, fish, nuts, some vegetables.
   - o **Supplementation**: Available as ubiquinone or ubiquinol supplements.

4. **Quercetin**:
   - o **Benefits**: Has antioxidant and anti-inflammatory properties, supports lung function, and reduces histamine release.
   - o **Sources**: Apples, onions, berries, and tea.
   - o **Supplementation**: Available in capsule or powder form.

Epicardium

The epicardium is the outermost layer of the heart's wall, playing a critical role in protecting the heart and contributing to its function. Here's a detailed look at the epicardium:

1. **Location**:
    - The epicardium is the outermost layer of the three layers of the heart wall, lying superficial to the myocardium (middle muscular layer) and the endocardium (innermost layer).
2. **Composition**:
    - **Mesothelium**: The outermost layer is composed of a single layer of flat epithelial cells called mesothelial cells, which secrete a small amount of lubricating fluid.
    - **Connective Tissue**: Beneath the mesothelium is a layer of connective tissue, including collagen fibers, elastic fibers, and adipose tissue. This layer contains blood vessels, nerves, and lymphatics that supply the heart.
3. **Pericardium**:

- The epicardium is often considered part of the visceral layer of the serous pericardium, a double-walled sac that encloses the heart. The parietal layer of the serous pericardium lines the fibrous pericardium, which is the tough outer sac.

Functions

1. **Protection:**
   - The epicardium serves as a protective barrier for the heart, reducing friction between the heart and surrounding structures as the heart beats.
2. **Secretion of Pericardial Fluid:**
   - The mesothelial cells of the epicardium secrete a small amount of serous fluid into the pericardial cavity, providing lubrication and allowing smooth, frictionless movement of the heart within the pericardial sac.
3. **Fat Storage:**
   - The connective tissue layer contains adipose tissue, which stores fat and provides

cushioning and insulation for the heart.

4. **Vascular Supply**:
   - The epicardium contains blood vessels (including coronary arteries and veins) that supply oxygen and nutrients to the heart muscle and remove waste products.
5. **Nervous and Lymphatic Supply**:
   - Nerves within the epicardium help regulate heart function, while lymphatic vessels help drain excess fluid and protect against infections.

Development and Changes

1. **Embryonic Development**:
   - The epicardium develops from a structure called the proepicardial organ during embryogenesis. Cells from this organ migrate to the surface of the heart and differentiate into the various components of the epicardium.
2. **Aging and Disease**:
   - With aging and certain cardiovascular diseases, the epicardium can undergo changes

such as increased fat deposition, fibrosis (scarring), and inflammation. These changes can impact heart function and contribute to conditions like coronary artery disease.

Herbs, Vitamins, Minerals, and Supplements for Epicardium Health

To support the health of the epicardium and overall heart function, various natural remedies can be beneficial:

Herbs

1. **Turmeric:**
   - **Benefits**: Contains curcumin, which has anti-inflammatory and antioxidant properties that help protect heart tissues.
   - **Usage**: Used in cooking or taken as a supplement.
2. **Ginger:**
   - **Benefits**: Acts as an anti-inflammatory and antioxidant, helping to reduce oxidative stress and inflammation in the heart.

- **Usage**: Consumed fresh, as a tea, or in supplement form.

Vitamins

1. **Vitamin E**:
   - **Benefits**: Acts as an antioxidant, protecting the epicardium and other heart tissues from oxidative damage.
   - **Sources**: Nuts, seeds, spinach, and broccoli.
   - **Supplementation**: Available in capsule or liquid form.
2. **Vitamin C**:
   - **Benefits**: Supports collagen production, which is important for the structural integrity of the epicardium, and has antioxidant properties.
   - **Sources**: Citrus fruits, berries, bell peppers, broccoli.
   - **Supplementation**: Commonly taken as ascorbic acid supplements.

Minerals

1. **Magnesium**:

- o **Benefits**: Essential for muscle function, including the heart, and helps regulate heart rhythm.
  - o **Sources**: Nuts, seeds, whole grains, leafy green vegetables.
  - o **Supplementation**: Available as magnesium citrate, magnesium oxide, and other forms.
2. **Zinc**:
  - o **Benefits**: Supports immune function and helps in tissue repair and maintenance, including heart tissues.
  - o **Sources**: Meat, shellfish, legumes, seeds.
  - o **Supplementation**: Often taken as zinc gluconate or zinc citrate supplements.

Supplements

1. **Coenzyme Q10 (CoQ10)**:
  - o **Benefits**: Supports energy production in heart cells, reduces oxidative stress, and improves heart function.
  - o **Sources**: Meat, fish, nuts, some vegetables.

- **Supplementation**: Available as ubiquinone or ubiquinol supplements.

2. **Omega-3 Fatty Acids**:
   - **Benefits**: Reduce inflammation, support cardiovascular health, and protect against heart disease.
   - **Sources**: Fatty fish (salmon, mackerel), flaxseeds, chia seeds.
   - **Supplementation**: Commonly taken as fish oil or flaxseed oil supplements.

Myocardium

The myocardium is the thick, muscular middle layer of the heart wall, responsible for the contractile function that pumps blood throughout the body. Here's a detailed examination of the myocardium:

1. **Location:**
   - The myocardium is sandwiched between the epicardium (outer layer) and the endocardium (inner layer) of the heart wall.
2. **Composition:**
   - **Cardiac Muscle Cells (Cardiomyocytes):** The primary cell type in the myocardium, specialized for contraction. Cardiomyocytes are striated and branched, with a single central nucleus. They are connected by intercalated discs that facilitate synchronized contraction.
   - **Intercalated Discs:** Specialized junctions between cardiomyocytes that contain gap junctions and desmosomes, allowing for efficient

transmission of electrical
impulses and mechanical forces.

- **Extracellular Matrix**: A
  network of collagen and elastin
  fibers that provide structural
  support and elasticity to the
  myocardium.

3. **Layers of the Myocardium**:
   - **Subendocardial Layer**: The
     inner portion, adjacent to the
     endocardium, contains fewer
     muscle fibers and more
     connective tissue.
   - **Middle Layer**: The thickest
     portion, consisting mainly of
     cardiomyocytes arranged in a
     spiral pattern, allowing the heart
     to contract efficiently.
   - **Subepicardial Layer**: The
     outer portion, adjacent to the
     epicardium, contains a mix of
     muscle fibers and connective
     tissue.

Functions

1. **Contraction and Pumping**:
   - The primary function of the
     myocardium is to contract and
     generate the force needed to

pump blood through the heart's chambers and into the circulatory system. The coordinated contraction of cardiomyocytes ensures efficient blood flow.

2. **Electrical Conduction**:
   - The myocardium plays a critical role in the heart's electrical conduction system. The synchronized contraction of cardiomyocytes is controlled by electrical impulses generated by the sinoatrial (SA) node and conducted through the atrioventricular (AV) node and the Purkinje fibers.

3. **Adaptation and Remodeling**:
   - The myocardium can adapt to increased workload by hypertrophy (increasing the size of cardiomyocytes) and remodeling its structure in response to chronic stress, such as high blood pressure or heart disease.

Blood Supply

1. **Coronary Arteries**:

- The myocardium receives oxygen-rich blood from the coronary arteries, which branch off from the aorta. The main coronary arteries are the left coronary artery (which divides into the left anterior descending and circumflex arteries) and the right coronary artery.

2. **Coronary Veins**:
   - Deoxygenated blood is drained from the myocardium by the coronary veins, which empty into the coronary sinus and then into the right atrium.

3. **Capillary Network**:
   - An extensive network of capillaries ensures that every cardiomyocyte receives adequate oxygen and nutrients, while waste products are efficiently removed.

Pathophysiology

1. **Ischemia and Infarction**:
   - Reduced blood flow to the myocardium, often due to coronary artery disease, can lead to ischemia (insufficient oxygen supply) and myocardial infarction

(heart attack), causing damage or death of cardiomyocytes.

2. **Cardiomyopathies**:
   - Diseases that affect the myocardium, such as hypertrophic cardiomyopathy (thickened myocardium) and dilated cardiomyopathy (enlarged heart chambers), can impair the heart's ability to pump blood effectively.

3. **Heart Failure**:
   - Progressive weakening of the myocardium, due to various conditions, can lead to heart failure, where the heart cannot pump sufficient blood to meet the body's needs.

The myocardium is a vital component of the heart, responsible for the contractile force that drives blood circulation. Its complex structure, specialized cells, and efficient blood supply are essential for maintaining cardiovascular health and function. Understanding the myocardium's role and potential pathologies is crucial for diagnosing and treating heart conditions effectively.

Herbs, Vitamins, Minerals, and Supplements for Myocardial Health

Supporting the myocardium, or heart muscle, is crucial for maintaining optimal cardiovascular function. Here are some alternative herbs, vitamins, minerals, and supplements that can help support, maintain, and heal the myocardium.

Herbs

1. **Cayenne Pepper**:
   - **Benefits**: Enhances blood flow, reduces blood pressure, and has anti-inflammatory properties.
   - **Usage**: Can be added to food, taken as a tincture, or in capsule form.
2. **Astragalus**:
   - **Benefits**: Strengthens the immune system, reduces inflammation, and improves heart function.
   - **Usage**: Typically used as a tea, tincture, or in capsule form.
3. **Bilberry**:
   - **Benefits**: Rich in antioxidants, improves circulation, and supports blood vessel health.

- o **Usage**: Consumed as dried berries, tea, or in supplement form.

4. **Reishi Mushroom**:
   - o **Benefits**: Reduces inflammation, supports immune function, and has cardioprotective effects.
   - o **Usage**: Available as a powder, tincture, or in capsule form.

Vitamins

1. **Vitamin D**:
   - o **Benefits**: Supports cardiovascular health, helps regulate blood pressure, and reduces inflammation.
   - o **Sources**: Sun exposure, fortified foods, fatty fish.
   - o **Supplementation**: Available as vitamin D3 supplements.
2. **Vitamin K2**:
   - o **Benefits**: Helps direct calcium to bones and away from arteries, reducing arterial calcification.
   - o **Sources**: Fermented foods (natto), dairy products, green leafy vegetables.

- 　○ **Supplementation**: Often found in K2 supplements (MK-7 form).
3. **Vitamin B12**:
   - ○ **Benefits**: Essential for red blood cell production and reducing homocysteine levels, which can affect heart health.
   - ○ **Sources**: Meat, fish, dairy products, fortified cereals.
   - ○ **Supplementation**: Available as cyanocobalamin or methylcobalamin supplements.

Minerals

1. **Selenium**:
   - ○ **Benefits**: Acts as an antioxidant, protecting heart cells from oxidative damage.
   - ○ **Sources**: Brazil nuts, seafood, organ meats.
   - ○ **Supplementation**: Available in forms like selenium selenite or selenomethionine.
2. **Copper**:
   - ○ **Benefits**: Essential for the formation of red blood cells and maintaining healthy blood vessels.

- **Sources**: Shellfish, nuts, seeds, whole grains.
  - **Supplementation**: Commonly found in multivitamins or as standalone supplements.

3. **Chromium**:
   - **Benefits**: Helps regulate blood sugar levels, which is important for heart health.
   - **Sources**: Broccoli, grape juice, whole grains, lean meats.
   - **Supplementation**: Available in forms like chromium picolinate or chromium polynicotinate.

Supplements

1. **Alpha-Lipoic Acid (ALA)**:
   - **Benefits**: Acts as an antioxidant, reduces inflammation, and supports mitochondrial function in heart cells.
   - **Sources**: Spinach, broccoli, potatoes.
   - **Supplementation**: Available as capsules or tablets.
2. **Resveratrol**:
   - **Benefits**: Has antioxidant and anti-inflammatory properties, supports blood vessel health, and

improves cardiovascular
function.

- o **Sources**: Red grapes, red wine, berries.
- o **Supplementation**: Available in capsule or tablet form.

3. **D-Ribose**:
   - o **Benefits**: Supports energy production in heart cells and improves heart muscle function.
   - o **Sources**: Naturally occurring in small amounts in food.
   - o **Supplementation**: Available in powder or capsule form.
4. **L-Arginine**:
   - o **Benefits**: Helps produce nitric oxide, which relaxes blood vessels and improves blood flow.
   - o **Sources**: Meat, poultry, fish, dairy.
   - o **Supplementation**: Available in powder or capsule form.

Endocardium

The endocardium is the thin, innermost layer of the heart wall, lining the interior of the heart chambers and covering the heart valves. It plays a critical role in maintaining the heart's structure and function.

1. **Location**:
     o   The endocardium lines the inner surface of the heart chambers, including the atria and ventricles, and extends over the heart valves.
2. **Composition**:
     o   **Endothelial Cells**: The inner surface of the endocardium is composed of a single layer of endothelial cells, which are flat, smooth cells that provide a slick, friction-reducing surface for blood flow.
     o   **Subendothelial Layer**: Beneath the endothelial cells lies the subendothelial layer, made up of loose connective tissue, collagen fibers, elastin fibers, and fibroblasts. This layer provides structural support and elasticity.
     o   **Myoelastic Layer**: Contains smooth muscle cells and elastic

fibers, which contribute to the flexibility and resilience of the heart wall.
  - **Subendocardial Layer**: The outermost layer of the endocardium, adjacent to the myocardium, contains connective tissue, small blood vessels, and Purkinje fibers (specialized conductive fibers involved in the heart's electrical conduction system).

Functions

1. **Smooth Surface for Blood Flow:**
   - The endocardium provides a smooth, frictionless surface that minimizes resistance to blood flow within the heart chambers and over the heart valves.
2. **Barrier Function**:
   - Acts as a barrier between the blood in the heart chambers and the myocardium, preventing the infiltration of blood cells and pathogens into the heart muscle.
3. **Regulation of Contraction**:
   - The subendocardial layer contains Purkinje fibers, which

are part of the heart's electrical conduction system. These fibers help transmit electrical impulses rapidly, ensuring coordinated contraction of the heart muscle.

4. **Valve Function**:
    o   The endocardium extends over the heart valves, contributing to their structure and function. It helps maintain valve integrity and ensures proper closure during the cardiac cycle to prevent backflow of blood.

Blood Supply

1. **Microcirculation**:
    o   The endocardium is supplied by a network of small blood vessels that originate from the coronary arteries. This microcirculation ensures the endocardium receives adequate oxygen and nutrients.
2. **Nutrient Diffusion**:
    o   In addition to direct blood supply, nutrients and oxygen diffuse from the blood in the heart chambers through the endocardial layer to reach the cells.

Pathophysiology

1. **Endocarditis**:
   - An infection of the endocardium, typically caused by bacteria, can lead to inflammation and damage to the heart valves. This condition, known as endocarditis, can result in serious complications, including heart failure and systemic embolism.
2. **Valvular Heart Disease**:
   - Diseases affecting the endocardial layer of the heart valves can lead to valvular stenosis (narrowing) or regurgitation (leakage), impairing the heart's ability to pump blood efficiently.
3. **Fibrosis and Thickening**:
   - Chronic inflammation or other pathological conditions can cause fibrosis (thickening) of the endocardium, which may interfere with normal heart function and increase the risk of arrhythmias.

The endocardium is a vital layer of the heart, playing crucial roles in maintaining a smooth blood flow, protecting the heart muscle, and ensuring proper valve function. Understanding its structure and function is essential for diagnosing and treating heart conditions that affect the endocardium.

Herbs, Vitamins, Minerals, and Supplements for Endocardial Health

Supporting the health of the endocardium, the innermost layer of the heart wall, is essential for overall cardiovascular function. Here are some herbs, vitamins, minerals, and supplements that can help support, maintain, and heal the endocardium.

Herbs

1. **Turmeric:**
    - **Benefits**: Contains curcumin, which has anti-inflammatory and antioxidant properties that protect the heart and reduce inflammation in the endocardium.
    - **Usage**: Can be used as a spice in food, taken as a tea, or in capsule form.
2. **Ginger:**

- **Benefits**: Has anti-inflammatory effects, helps improve circulation, and reduces oxidative stress on heart tissues.
  - **Usage**: Fresh ginger can be added to food, taken as a tea, or in supplement form.
3. **Olive Leaf**:
  - **Benefits**: Has antimicrobial and anti-inflammatory properties, which can help prevent infections such as endocarditis.
  - **Usage**: Available as a tea, tincture, or in capsule form.
4. **Holy Basil**:
  - **Benefits**: Reduces stress and inflammation, supporting overall heart health and endocardial function.
  - **Usage**: Often used as a tea, tincture, or in capsule form.

Vitamins

1. **Vitamin A**:
  - **Benefits**: Supports immune function and has antioxidant properties that protect the endocardium from oxidative stress.

o **Sources**: Carrots, sweet potatoes, spinach, and dairy products.
o **Supplementation**: Available in retinol or beta-carotene supplements.

2. **Vitamin B9 (Folate)**:
   o **Benefits**: Reduces homocysteine levels, which can lower the risk of cardiovascular diseases affecting the endocardium.
   o **Sources**: Leafy green vegetables, legumes, nuts, and fortified cereals.
   o **Supplementation**: Commonly found in B-complex vitamins or as standalone folic acid supplements.

3. **Vitamin B3 (Niacin)**:
   o **Benefits**: Helps improve blood lipid levels, supporting cardiovascular health and endocardial function.
   o **Sources**: Meat, fish, poultry, and fortified grains.
   o **Supplementation**: Available as nicotinic acid or niacinamide supplements.

Minerals

1. **Zinc:**
   - **Benefits**: Essential for immune function and helps repair tissues, including the endocardium.
   - **Sources**: Meat, shellfish, legumes, seeds, and nuts.
   - **Supplementation**: Available in forms such as zinc gluconate or zinc citrate.
2. **Manganese:**
   - **Benefits**: Supports antioxidant enzymes that protect heart tissues from oxidative damage.
   - **Sources**: Whole grains, nuts, leafy vegetables, and teas.
   - **Supplementation**: Often found in multivitamins or as standalone supplements.
3. **Iron:**
   - **Benefits**: Essential for oxygen transport in the blood, supporting overall cardiovascular function.
   - **Sources**: Red meat, poultry, fish, lentils, and spinach.
   - **Supplementation**: Available as ferrous sulfate, ferrous gluconate, or other forms.

Supplements

1. **N-Acetyl Cysteine (NAC):**
   - **Benefits**: Boosts levels of glutathione, a powerful antioxidant that protects heart tissues, including the endocardium.
   - **Sources**: Found in small amounts in foods, primarily used as a supplement.
   - **Supplementation**: Available in capsule or powder form.
2. **Policosanol:**
   - **Benefits**: Helps improve blood lipid levels and supports overall cardiovascular health.
   - **Sources**: Derived from sugarcane, beeswax, and other sources.
   - **Supplementation**: Available in capsule or tablet form.
3. **Tocotrienols:**
   - **Benefits**: A form of vitamin E with potent antioxidant properties that protect the endocardium.

- **Sources**: Palm oil, rice bran oil, and barley.
    - **Supplementation**: Available as supplements specifically labeled as tocotrienols.
4. **Quercetin**:
    - **Benefits**: A flavonoid with anti-inflammatory and antioxidant properties, supporting heart health and protecting the endocardium.
    - **Sources**: Apples, onions, berries, and green tea.
    - **Supplementation**: Available in capsule or tablet form.

Right Atrium

The right atrium is one of the four chambers of the heart, playing a crucial role in the circulatory system. It receives deoxygenated blood from the body and pumps it into the right ventricle, which then sends it to the lungs for oxygenation.

1. **Location**:
   - The right atrium is located in the upper right portion of the heart, above the right ventricle and adjacent to the left atrium.
2. **Anatomical Features**:
   - **Auricle**: A small, ear-like extension that increases the atrial volume.
   - **Fossa Ovalis**: A depression in the interatrial septum, a remnant of the fetal foramen ovale.
   - **Crista Terminalis**: A smooth, muscular ridge in the atrium that separates the pectinate muscles from the smoother posterior wall.
   - **Pectinate Muscles**: Parallel ridges in the anterior wall of the right atrium that increase the atrial contraction force.
3. **Blood Inflow**:

- ○ **Superior Vena Cava (SVC)**: Brings deoxygenated blood from the upper body (head, neck, arms).
  - ○ **Inferior Vena Cava (IVC)**: Brings deoxygenated blood from the lower body (legs, abdomen).
  - ○ **Coronary Sinus**: Drains deoxygenated blood from the heart's own circulation.
4. **Blood Outflow**:
  - ○ Blood from the right atrium flows into the right ventricle through the tricuspid valve during atrial contraction.

Function

1. **Blood Reception**:
  - ○ The right atrium receives deoxygenated blood from the systemic circulation via the SVC and IVC, and from the coronary sinus, ensuring the continuous flow of blood to the heart for reoxygenation.
2. **Atrial Contraction**:
  - ○ During atrial systole (contraction), the right atrium contracts to push blood through

the tricuspid valve into the right ventricle, contributing to the overall cardiac output.

3. **Electrical Conduction**:
   - The right atrium houses the sinoatrial (SA) node, the heart's natural pacemaker, which initiates electrical impulses that regulate the heartbeat. These impulses travel through the atria to the atrioventricular (AV) node and into the ventricles.

Blood Supply

1. **Arterial Supply**:
   - The right atrium is supplied by branches of the right coronary artery, which provides oxygenated blood to the heart tissue.
2. **Venous Drainage**:
   - Deoxygenated blood from the right atrium drains into the right ventricle and is then pumped to the lungs for oxygenation.

Pathophysiology

1. **Atrial Fibrillation**:

- A common condition where the atria, including the right atrium, experience uncoordinated electrical activity, leading to irregular and often rapid heartbeats. This can reduce the efficiency of blood flow from the atrium to the ventricle.

2. **Atrial Septal Defect (ASD):**
   - A congenital condition where there is an opening in the interatrial septum, allowing blood to flow between the left and right atria. This can lead to increased blood flow to the right atrium and right ventricle, causing enlargement and potentially heart failure if untreated.

3. **Right Atrial Enlargement:**
   - Can result from conditions like pulmonary hypertension or tricuspid valve disorders. Enlargement of the right atrium can affect its function and lead to complications such as arrhythmias.

The right atrium plays a vital role in the heart's function, acting as a receiving chamber for deoxygenated blood from the body and a critical component in the heart's electrical conduction system. Understanding its structure and function is essential for diagnosing and managing various cardiovascular conditions.

Herbs, Vitamins, Minerals, and Supplements for Right Atrium Health

Supporting the health of the right atrium is crucial for maintaining overall cardiovascular function. Here are some herbs, vitamins, minerals, and supplements that can help support, maintain, and heal the right atrium.

Herbs

1. **Hawthorn Berry:**
   - **Benefits**: Enhances heart function, improves blood flow, and has cardioprotective effects.
   - **Usage**: Available as a tea, tincture, or in capsule form.
2. **Motherwort:**
   - **Benefits**: Has calming effects on the heart, helps reduce palpitations and arrhythmias,

and improves overall heart function.

- ○ **Usage**: Typically used as a tea or tincture.

3. **Garlic**:
   - ○ **Benefits**: Improves circulation, lowers blood pressure, and has anti-inflammatory and antioxidant properties.
   - ○ **Usage**: Can be consumed fresh, as an extract, or in capsule form.

4. **Arjuna**:
   - ○ **Benefits**: Traditional Ayurvedic herb known for strengthening heart muscles and improving cardiovascular function.
   - ○ **Usage**: Often taken as a powder or in capsule form.

Vitamins

1. **Vitamin C**:
   - ○ **Benefits**: Acts as an antioxidant, supports blood vessel health, and reduces inflammation.
   - ○ **Sources**: Citrus fruits, strawberries, bell peppers, broccoli.

- **Supplementation**: Available as ascorbic acid in tablets, capsules, or powder form.

2. **Vitamin E**:
   - **Benefits**: Protects heart tissues from oxidative damage and supports immune function.
   - **Sources**: Nuts, seeds, spinach, and vegetable oils.
   - **Supplementation**: Available as tocopherol in capsules or tablets.

3. **Vitamin B6**:
   - **Benefits**: Helps regulate homocysteine levels, reducing the risk of cardiovascular disease.
   - **Sources**: Fish, poultry, potatoes, chickpeas, and bananas.
   - **Supplementation**: Commonly found in B-complex vitamins or as standalone pyridoxine supplements.

Minerals

1. **Magnesium**:
   - **Benefits**: Essential for heart muscle function, helps maintain normal heart rhythm, and reduces blood pressure.

- **Sources**: Nuts, seeds, green leafy vegetables, whole grains.
  - **Supplementation**: Available as magnesium citrate, glycinate, or oxide.

2. **Potassium**:
   - **Benefits**: Helps regulate heartbeats and fluid balance, and lowers blood pressure.
   - **Sources**: Bananas, oranges, potatoes, and spinach.
   - **Supplementation**: Available in forms like potassium gluconate or citrate.

3. **Calcium**:
   - **Benefits**: Essential for muscle contractions, including the heart, and helps maintain a regular heartbeat.
   - **Sources**: Dairy products, leafy greens, and fortified foods.
   - **Supplementation**: Often found in calcium carbonate or citrate supplements.

Supplements

1. **Coenzyme Q10 (CoQ10)**:
   - **Benefits**: Supports mitochondrial function, improves

heart muscle energy production, and acts as an antioxidant.

- o **Sources**: Found in small amounts in meat and fish.
- o **Supplementation**: Available in ubiquinone or ubiquinol form.

2. **Omega-3 Fatty Acids**:
   - o **Benefits**: Reduces inflammation, lowers triglyceride levels, and supports overall heart health.
   - o **Sources**: Fatty fish (salmon, mackerel), flaxseeds, chia seeds.
   - o **Supplementation**: Available as fish oil or flaxseed oil capsules.

3. **Taurine**:
   - o **Benefits**: Supports cardiovascular function, helps regulate calcium levels in heart cells, and improves blood flow.
   - o **Sources**: Meat, fish, dairy products.
   - o **Supplementation**: Available as capsules or powder.

4. **L-Carnitine**:
   - o **Benefits**: Supports energy production in heart cells, improves exercise tolerance, and

reduces symptoms of heart
failure.

- ○ **Sources**: Red meat, dairy
  products.
- ○ **Supplementation**: Available in
  acetyl-L-carnitine or L-carnitine
  tartrate form.

Right Ventricle

The right ventricle is one of the four chambers of the heart, playing a crucial role in the pulmonary circulation by pumping deoxygenated blood to the lungs for oxygenation.

1. **Location**:
   - The right ventricle is located in the lower right portion of the heart, beneath the right atrium and adjacent to the left ventricle.
2. **Anatomical Features**:
   - **Chamber Shape**: The right ventricle has a crescent shape in cross-section and is thinner-walled compared to the left ventricle.
   - **Trabeculae Carneae**: Irregular muscular ridges on the internal surface that increase the surface area and assist with contraction.
   - **Moderator Band**: A muscular band that contains part of the heart's conduction system, ensuring coordinated contraction of the right ventricle.
   - **Papillary Muscles**: Small muscle projections attached to

the tricuspid valve via chordae tendineae, helping to prevent valve prolapse during ventricular contraction.

- **Chordae Tendineae**: Tendinous cords that connect the papillary muscles to the tricuspid valve leaflets.

3. **Blood Inflow and Outflow**:
   - **Inflow**: Blood enters the right ventricle from the right atrium through the tricuspid valve.
   - **Outflow**: Blood is pumped from the right ventricle into the pulmonary trunk through the pulmonary valve, leading to the lungs for oxygenation.

Function

1. **Blood Pumping**:
   - The right ventricle receives deoxygenated blood from the right atrium and pumps it into the pulmonary arteries, which transport it to the lungs for oxygenation.
2. **Valve Function**:
   - The tricuspid valve ensures one-way blood flow from the

right atrium to the right ventricle,
while the pulmonary valve
prevents backflow of blood from
the pulmonary trunk into the
right ventricle.

3. **Electrical Conduction**:
    - The right ventricle is part of the
      heart's conduction system,
      receiving electrical impulses that
      trigger synchronized contraction,
      facilitating efficient blood
      ejection.

Blood Supply

1. **Arterial Supply**:
    - The right ventricle is primarily
      supplied by branches of the right
      coronary artery, providing
      oxygenated blood to the heart
      muscle.
2. **Venous Drainage**:
    - Deoxygenated blood from the
      right ventricle is collected by
      cardiac veins and drains into the
      right atrium via the coronary
      sinus.

Pathophysiology

1. **Right Ventricular Hypertrophy (RVH):**
   - Thickening of the right ventricular wall, often due to conditions like pulmonary hypertension or chronic lung disease, increasing the workload on the right ventricle.
2. **Right Ventricular Failure:**
   - Occurs when the right ventricle cannot pump blood efficiently, leading to symptoms such as fluid retention, swelling, and shortness of breath. It can be caused by conditions like left-sided heart failure, pulmonary hypertension, or congenital heart defects.
3. **Tricuspid Valve Disorders:**
   - Diseases affecting the tricuspid valve, such as tricuspid regurgitation or stenosis, can impair right ventricular function and lead to right-sided heart failure.
4. **Pulmonary Valve Disorders:**
   - Conditions like pulmonary valve stenosis or regurgitation can impact blood flow from the right

ventricle to the lungs, affecting overall cardiovascular function.

The right ventricle plays a vital role in pulmonary circulation, ensuring that deoxygenated blood is efficiently pumped to the lungs for oxygenation. Understanding its structure and function is essential for diagnosing and managing various cardiovascular conditions that affect the right ventricle.

Herbs, Vitamins, Minerals, and Supplements for Right Ventricle Health

Supporting the health of the right ventricle is essential for maintaining overall cardiovascular function. Here are some herbs, vitamins, minerals, and supplements that can help support, maintain, and heal the right ventricle.

Herbs

1. **Astragalus**:
    - **Benefits**: Strengthens the heart, improves circulation, and has anti-inflammatory properties.

o   **Usage**: Typically used as a tea,
        tincture, or in capsule form.

2. **Reishi Mushroom**:
   o   **Benefits**: Supports heart health,
       enhances immune function, and
       reduces inflammation.
   o   **Usage**: Available as a tea,
       extract, or in capsule form.

3. **Dandelion**:
   o   **Benefits**: Acts as a diuretic,
       reducing fluid buildup and easing
       the burden on the heart.
   o   **Usage**: Consumed as a tea,
       tincture, or in capsule form.

4. **Ginkgo Biloba**:
   o   **Benefits**: Improves blood flow,
       acts as an antioxidant, and
       supports overall heart health.
   o   **Usage**: Available in capsule,
       tablet, or tea form.

Vitamins

1. **Vitamin B12**:
   o   **Benefits**: Supports red blood
       cell production and
       cardiovascular health, reduces
       homocysteine levels.
   o   **Sources**: Meat, dairy, and
       fortified cereals.

- o **Supplementation**: Available as cyanocobalamin or methylcobalamin in tablets, capsules, or injections.

2. **Vitamin D**:
   - o **Benefits**: Supports heart muscle function and reduces the risk of cardiovascular disease.
   - o **Sources**: Sunlight exposure, fatty fish, fortified dairy products.
   - o **Supplementation**: Available as cholecalciferol (D3) or ergocalciferol (D2) in tablets, capsules, or liquid form.

3. **Vitamin K2**:
   - o **Benefits**: Helps regulate calcium deposition, supporting vascular health and reducing arterial calcification.
   - o **Sources**: Fermented foods like natto, dairy, and meat.
   - o **Supplementation**: Available as menaquinone in tablets or capsules.

Minerals

1. **Zinc**:
   - o **Benefits**: Supports immune function, reduces inflammation,

and is crucial for overall heart health.

- ○ **Sources**: Meat, shellfish, legumes, seeds, and nuts.
- ○ **Supplementation**: Available as zinc gluconate, citrate, or picolinate in tablets or capsules.

2. **Selenium**:
   - ○ **Benefits**: Acts as an antioxidant, protects heart cells from oxidative damage, and supports immune function.
   - ○ **Sources**: Brazil nuts, fish, eggs, and whole grains.
   - ○ **Supplementation**: Available as selenomethionine or selenium yeast in tablets or capsules.

3. **Copper**:
   - ○ **Benefits**: Necessary for heart and blood vessel health, aids in iron absorption, and supports immune function.
   - ○ **Sources**: Shellfish, seeds, nuts, and whole grains.
   - ○ **Supplementation**: Available as copper gluconate or sulfate in tablets or capsules.

Supplements

1. **L-Arginine**:
   - **Benefits**: An amino acid that helps produce nitric oxide, improving blood flow and reducing blood pressure.
   - **Sources**: Meat, dairy, and legumes.
   - **Supplementation**: Available as powder or capsules.
2. **Resveratrol**:
   - **Benefits**: Found in red wine and grapes, it has antioxidant properties that support heart health and reduce inflammation.
   - **Sources**: Red grapes, red wine, berries.
   - **Supplementation**: Available in capsule or tablet form.
3. **N-Acetylcysteine (NAC)**:
   - **Benefits**: Acts as an antioxidant, supports respiratory health, and enhances heart function.
   - **Sources**: Not commonly found in foods.
   - **Supplementation**: Available in capsule or tablet form.
4. **Taurine**:

- **Benefits**: Supports cardiovascular function, helps regulate calcium levels in heart cells, and improves blood flow.
- **Sources**: Meat, fish, dairy products.
- **Supplementation**: Available as capsules or powder.

Left Atrium

The left atrium is one of the four chambers of the heart, playing a vital role in receiving oxygenated blood from the lungs and pumping it into the left ventricle, which then distributes it throughout the body.

1. **Location**:
    - The left atrium is located in the upper left portion of the heart, above the left ventricle and adjacent to the right atrium.
2. **Anatomical Features**:
    - **Auricle**: A small, ear-like extension that increases the atrial volume and helps to store blood.
    - **Pulmonary Veins**: Four veins (two from each lung) that deliver oxygenated blood from the lungs to the left atrium.
    - **Interatrial Septum**: The wall that separates the left atrium from the right atrium, containing the fossa ovalis, a remnant of the fetal foramen ovale.
    - **Smooth Inner Wall**: Unlike the right atrium, the inner wall of the left atrium is smooth and lacks

pectinate muscles, except in the
auricle.

3. **Blood Inflow**:
   - The left atrium receives
     oxygenated blood from the lungs
     through the pulmonary veins.

4. **Blood Outflow**:
   - Blood from the left atrium flows
     into the left ventricle through the
     mitral (bicuspid) valve during
     atrial contraction.

Function

1. **Blood Reception**:
   - The left atrium receives
     oxygen-rich blood from the lungs
     and serves as a holding chamber
     before transferring it to the left
     ventricle.

2. **Atrial Contraction**:
   - During atrial systole, the left
     atrium contracts to push blood
     through the mitral valve into the
     left ventricle, contributing to the
     efficient pumping of blood to the
     body.

3. **Electrical Conduction**:
   - The left atrium participates in the
     heart's electrical conduction

system, receiving impulses from the sinoatrial (SA) node, which coordinates the contraction of the atria and ventricles.

Blood Supply

1. **Arterial Supply**:
    - The left atrium is supplied by branches of the left coronary artery, specifically the circumflex artery, which provides oxygenated blood to the atrial myocardium.
2. **Venous Drainage**:
    - Deoxygenated blood from the left atrium is collected by small cardiac veins and drains into the right atrium via the coronary sinus.

Pathophysiology

1. **Atrial Fibrillation**:
    - A common arrhythmia where the atria, including the left atrium, experience rapid and irregular electrical activity, leading to ineffective atrial contraction and an increased risk of stroke due to blood clot formation.

2. **Mitral Valve Disorders**:
   - Conditions such as mitral valve stenosis or regurgitation can impede blood flow from the left atrium to the left ventricle, causing increased atrial pressure and enlargement, potentially leading to atrial fibrillation and heart failure.
3. **Left Atrial Enlargement**:
   - Can result from chronic conditions like hypertension or mitral valve disease, leading to increased atrial pressure and volume, which can impair the atrial function and increase the risk of arrhythmias.
4. **Pulmonary Hypertension**:
   - Elevated pressure in the pulmonary arteries can lead to increased workload on the left atrium, contributing to left atrial enlargement and dysfunction.

The left atrium is essential for efficient cardiac function, ensuring that oxygenated blood from the lungs is properly transferred to the left ventricle for systemic distribution. Understanding its structure, function, and associated pathologies is crucial for diagnosing and managing cardiovascular conditions that affect the left atrium.

Herbs, Vitamins, Minerals, and Supplements for Left Atrium Health

Maintaining the health of the left atrium is crucial for optimal cardiovascular function. Here are some herbs, vitamins, minerals, and supplements that can help support, maintain, and heal the left atrium.

Herbs

1. **Bilberry:**
   - **Benefits**: Rich in antioxidants, supports blood vessel health, and improves circulation.
   - **Usage**: Available as a tea, tincture, or in capsule form.
2. **Olive Leaf:**
   - **Benefits**: Improves cardiovascular health, lowers blood pressure, and has anti-inflammatory properties.
   - **Usage**: Typically used as an extract or in capsule form.
3. **Linden Flower:**

- ○ **Benefits**: Calms the heart, reduces anxiety, and helps with hypertension.
  - ○ **Usage**: Commonly consumed as a tea or tincture.
4. **Hibiscus**:
   - ○ **Benefits**: Lowers blood pressure, acts as an antioxidant, and supports heart health.
   - ○ **Usage**: Available as a tea or in capsule form.

Vitamins

1. **Vitamin B1 (Thiamine)**:
   - ○ **Benefits**: Supports energy production in heart cells, reduces the risk of heart disease.
   - ○ **Sources**: Whole grains, pork, legumes, and seeds.
   - ○ **Supplementation**: Available as thiamine mononitrate or hydrochloride in tablets or capsules.
2. **Vitamin B9 (Folate)**:
   - ○ **Benefits**: Helps regulate homocysteine levels, reducing the risk of cardiovascular disease.
   - ○ **Sources**: Leafy greens, legumes, and fortified cereals.

- **Supplementation**: Available as folic acid or methylfolate in tablets or capsules.

3. **Vitamin C**:
   - **Benefits**: Supports collagen synthesis, improves blood vessel health, and acts as an antioxidant.
   - **Sources**: Citrus fruits, berries, bell peppers, and broccoli.
   - **Supplementation**: Available as ascorbic acid in tablets, capsules, or powder form.

Minerals

1. **Magnesium**:
   - **Benefits**: Essential for heart muscle function, helps maintain normal heart rhythm, and reduces blood pressure.
   - **Sources**: Nuts, seeds, green leafy vegetables, whole grains.
   - **Supplementation**: Available as magnesium citrate, glycinate, or oxide.

2. **Potassium**:
   - **Benefits**: Helps regulate heartbeats and fluid balance, and lowers blood pressure.

- ○ **Sources**: Bananas, oranges, potatoes, and spinach.
  - ○ **Supplementation**: Available in forms like potassium gluconate or citrate.
3. **Calcium**:
   - ○ **Benefits**: Essential for muscle contractions, including the heart, and helps maintain a regular heartbeat.
   - ○ **Sources**: Dairy products, leafy greens, and fortified foods.
   - ○ **Supplementation**: Often found in calcium carbonate or citrate supplements.

Supplements

1. **L-Carnitine**:
   - ○ **Benefits**: Supports energy production in heart cells, improves exercise tolerance, and reduces symptoms of heart failure.
   - ○ **Sources**: Red meat, dairy products.
   - ○ **Supplementation**: Available in acetyl-L-carnitine or L-carnitine tartrate form.
2. **Taurine**:

o   **Benefits**: Supports cardiovascular function, helps regulate calcium levels in heart cells, and improves blood flow.
   o   **Sources**: Meat, fish, dairy products.
   o   **Supplementation**: Available as capsules or powder.
3. **Coenzyme Q10 (CoQ10)**:
   o   **Benefits**: Supports mitochondrial function, improves heart muscle energy production, and acts as an antioxidant.
   o   **Sources**: Found in small amounts in meat and fish.
   o   **Supplementation**: Available in ubiquinone or ubiquinol form.
4. **Omega-3 Fatty Acids**:
   o   **Benefits**: Reduces inflammation, lowers triglyceride levels, and supports overall heart health.
   o   **Sources**: Fatty fish (salmon, mackerel), flaxseeds, chia seeds.
   o   **Supplementation**: Available as fish oil or flaxseed oil capsules.

Left Ventricle

The left ventricle is one of the four chambers of the heart, responsible for pumping oxygenated blood into the systemic circulation through the aorta. It plays a crucial role in maintaining adequate blood flow and pressure throughout the body.

1. **Location**:
   - The left ventricle is located in the lower left portion of the heart, below the left atrium and adjacent to the right ventricle.
2. **Anatomical Features**:
   - **Chamber Shape**: The left ventricle has a conical shape and is thicker-walled compared to the right ventricle due to the higher pressure it needs to generate to pump blood throughout the body.
   - **Papillary Muscles**: Small muscle projections attached to the mitral valve via chordae tendineae, which help prevent valve prolapse during ventricular contraction.
   - **Chordae Tendineae**: Tendinous cords that connect the papillary muscles to the mitral

valve leaflets, ensuring proper
valve function.

- o **Trabeculae Carneae**: Irregular
  muscular ridges on the internal
  surface that increase the surface
  area and assist with contraction.

3. **Blood Inflow and Outflow**:
   - o **Inflow**: Blood enters the left
     ventricle from the left atrium
     through the mitral (bicuspid)
     valve.
   - o **Outflow**: Blood is pumped from
     the left ventricle into the aorta
     through the aortic valve, leading
     to the systemic circulation.

Function

1. **Blood Pumping**:
   - o The left ventricle receives
     oxygenated blood from the left
     atrium and pumps it into the
     aorta, distributing it to the entire
     body.

2. **Valve Function**:
   - o The mitral valve ensures one-way
     blood flow from the left atrium to
     the left ventricle, while the aortic
     valve prevents backflow of blood

from the aorta into the left
ventricle.

3. **Electrical Conduction**:
   - The left ventricle is part of the heart's conduction system, receiving electrical impulses that trigger synchronized contraction, facilitating efficient blood ejection.

Blood Supply

1. **Arterial Supply**:
   - The left ventricle is primarily supplied by branches of the left coronary artery, including the left anterior descending artery and the circumflex artery, providing oxygenated blood to the heart muscle.
2. **Venous Drainage**:
   - Deoxygenated blood from the left ventricle is collected by cardiac veins and drains into the right atrium via the coronary sinus.

Pathophysiology

1. **Left Ventricular Hypertrophy (LVH)**:
   - Thickening of the left ventricular wall, often due to conditions like

hypertension or aortic stenosis, increasing the workload on the left ventricle.

2. **Left Ventricular Failure**:
   - Occurs when the left ventricle cannot pump blood efficiently, leading to symptoms such as shortness of breath, fatigue, and fluid retention. It can be caused by conditions like myocardial infarction, cardiomyopathy, or valvular heart disease.

3. **Aortic Valve Disorders**:
   - Diseases affecting the aortic valve, such as aortic stenosis or regurgitation, can impair left ventricular function and lead to heart failure.

4. **Mitral Valve Disorders**:
   - Conditions like mitral regurgitation or stenosis can impede blood flow from the left atrium to the left ventricle, causing increased atrial pressure and left ventricular dysfunction.

The left ventricle plays a vital role in systemic circulation, ensuring that oxygenated blood is efficiently pumped to the entire body. Understanding its structure and function is essential for diagnosing and managing various cardiovascular conditions that affect the left ventricle.

Herbs, Vitamins, Minerals, and Supplements for Left Ventricle Health

Supporting the health of the left ventricle is essential for maintaining optimal cardiovascular function. Here are some herbs, vitamins, minerals, and supplements that can help support, maintain, and heal the left ventricle.

Herbs

1. **Hawthorn**:
    - **Benefits**: Strengthens the heart muscle, improves circulation, and reduces blood pressure.
    - **Usage**: Typically used as a tea, tincture, or in capsule form.
2. **Motherwort**:
    - **Benefits**: Supports heart health, reduces palpitations, and has a calming effect.

- **Usage**: Available as a tea, tincture, or in capsule form.

3. **Ginger**:
   - **Benefits**: Improves circulation, reduces inflammation, and supports cardiovascular health.
   - **Usage**: Consumed as a tea, extract, or in capsule form.

4. **Turmeric**:
   - **Benefits**: Contains curcumin, which has anti-inflammatory and antioxidant properties that support heart health.
   - **Usage**: Available as a spice, extract, or in capsule form.

Vitamins

1. **Vitamin E**:
   - **Benefits**: Acts as an antioxidant, supports heart health, and reduces oxidative stress.
   - **Sources**: Nuts, seeds, spinach, and broccoli.
   - **Supplementation**: Available as alpha-tocopherol in tablets or capsules.

2. **Vitamin B6**:
   - **Benefits**: Supports heart health by regulating homocysteine

levels, reducing the risk of cardiovascular disease.
  - ○ **Sources**: Poultry, fish, potatoes, and bananas.
  - ○ **Supplementation**: Available as pyridoxine in tablets or capsules.
3. **Vitamin B2 (Riboflavin)**:
  - ○ **Benefits**: Supports energy production in heart cells and maintains overall cardiovascular health.
  - ○ **Sources**: Dairy products, eggs, lean meats, and green leafy vegetables.
  - ○ **Supplementation**: Available as riboflavin in tablets or capsules.

Minerals

1. **Iron**:
  - ○ **Benefits**: Essential for oxygen transport in the blood, supports heart muscle function, and prevents anemia.
  - ○ **Sources**: Red meat, beans, spinach, and fortified cereals.
  - ○ **Supplementation**: Available as ferrous sulfate, gluconate, or fumarate.
2. **Chromium**:

- o **Benefits**: Helps regulate blood sugar levels, reducing the risk of heart disease.
  - o **Sources**: Broccoli, grape juice, potatoes, and whole grains.
  - o **Supplementation**: Available as chromium picolinate or chloride.
3. **Manganese**:
  - o **Benefits**: Supports heart health, acts as an antioxidant, and is essential for enzyme function.
  - o **Sources**: Nuts, seeds, whole grains, and leafy green vegetables.
  - o **Supplementation**: Available as manganese sulfate or gluconate.

Supplements

1. **Alpha-Lipoic Acid**:
  - o **Benefits**: Acts as an antioxidant, supports heart health, and improves mitochondrial function.
  - o **Sources**: Spinach, broccoli, and potatoes.
  - o **Supplementation**: Available in capsules or tablets.
2. **D-Ribose**:
  - o **Benefits**: Supports energy production in heart cells,

improves exercise tolerance, and enhances heart function.

  - **Sources**: Not commonly found in foods.
  - **Supplementation**: Available as powder or capsules.

3. **Polyphenols**:
  - **Benefits**: Found in foods like dark chocolate and green tea, they have antioxidant properties that support heart health and reduce inflammation.
  - **Sources**: Dark chocolate, green tea, berries.
  - **Supplementation**: Available in extract or capsule form.

4. **Magnesium Taurate**:
  - **Benefits**: Combines the benefits of magnesium and taurine, supporting heart function, reducing blood pressure, and improving circulation.
  - **Sources**: Not commonly found in foods.
  - **Supplementation**: Available in capsule form.

Tricuspid Valve

The tricuspid valve is one of the four main valves in the heart, playing a crucial role in regulating blood flow between the right atrium and the right ventricle. Its proper function is essential for maintaining unidirectional blood flow and preventing backflow within the heart.

1. **Location**:
   - The tricuspid valve is situated between the right atrium and the right ventricle.
2. **Anatomical Features**:
   - **Leaflets**: The valve has three cusps or leaflets—anterior, posterior, and septal—that open and close to regulate blood flow.
   - **Chordae Tendineae**: Tendinous cords connecting the leaflets to the papillary muscles, preventing the leaflets from prolapsing into the atrium during ventricular contraction.
   - **Papillary Muscles**: Small muscles within the right ventricle that anchor the chordae tendineae and aid in valve function.
3. **Function**:

- During atrial systole, the tricuspid valve opens, allowing blood to flow from the right atrium to the right ventricle. During ventricular systole, the valve closes to prevent backflow of blood into the right atrium.

Function

1. **Blood Flow Regulation**:
   - The tricuspid valve ensures unidirectional blood flow from the right atrium to the right ventricle, facilitating efficient circulation.
2. **Prevention of Backflow**:
   - By closing during ventricular contraction, the tricuspid valve prevents the backflow of blood into the right atrium, maintaining proper pressure and volume in the heart chambers.
3. **Synchronization with Heartbeat**:
   - The tricuspid valve opens and closes in coordination with the heart's electrical impulses, ensuring synchronized and efficient pumping action.

Blood Supply

1. **Arterial Supply**:
   - The tricuspid valve is supplied by the right coronary artery, which provides oxygenated blood to the valve tissue and surrounding structures.
2. **Venous Drainage**:
   - Deoxygenated blood from the tricuspid valve area drains into the right atrium via small cardiac veins.

Pathophysiology

1. **Tricuspid Valve Regurgitation**:
   - A condition where the valve does not close properly, allowing blood to flow back into the right atrium, leading to symptoms like fatigue, swelling, and atrial fibrillation.
2. **Tricuspid Valve Stenosis**:
   - Narrowing of the tricuspid valve opening, restricting blood flow from the right atrium to the right ventricle, causing increased atrial pressure and congestion.
3. **Infective Endocarditis**:

- o An infection of the tricuspid valve, often seen in intravenous drug users, which can cause valve damage and lead to regurgitation or stenosis.
4. **Congenital Defects**:
    - o Conditions like Ebstein's anomaly, where the tricuspid valve is malformed, leading to improper function and potential heart failure.

The tricuspid valve is essential for the proper functioning of the heart, ensuring that blood flows efficiently from the right atrium to the right ventricle and preventing backflow. Understanding its structure, function, and associated pathologies is crucial for diagnosing and managing conditions that affect this valve.

Herbs, Vitamins, Minerals, and Supplements for Tricuspid Valve Health

Maintaining the health of the tricuspid valve is vital for overall cardiovascular function. Here are some herbs, vitamins, minerals, and supplements that can help support, maintain, and heal the tricuspid valve.

Herbs

1. **Garlic:**
   - **Benefits**: Reduces inflammation, lowers blood pressure, and improves overall heart health.
   - **Usage**: Can be consumed raw, as an extract, or in capsule form.
2. **Ginkgo Biloba**:
   - **Benefits**: Enhances circulation, reduces blood clot formation, and provides antioxidant protection.
   - **Usage**: Available as a tea, tincture, or in capsule form.
3. **Green Tea**:
   - **Benefits**: Contains polyphenols that support heart health, reduce inflammation, and improve endothelial function.
   - **Usage**: Commonly consumed as a beverage or in capsule form.
4. **Cayenne Pepper**:
   - **Benefits**: Improves circulation, supports heart health, and has anti-inflammatory properties.

- Usage: Can be used as a spice, in extract form, or in capsules.

Vitamins

1. **Vitamin D**:
   - **Benefits**: Supports heart health, reduces inflammation, and helps regulate blood pressure.
   - **Sources**: Sunlight, fatty fish, fortified dairy products, and eggs.
   - **Supplementation**: Available as cholecalciferol (D3) in tablets or capsules.
2. **Vitamin K2**:
   - **Benefits**: Directs calcium to bones and away from arteries, preventing calcification and supporting cardiovascular health.
   - **Sources**: Fermented foods, cheese, and natto.
   - **Supplementation**: Available as menaquinone-7 (MK-7) in capsules.
3. **Vitamin B12**:
   - **Benefits**: Supports red blood cell formation and helps maintain proper cardiovascular function.
   - **Sources**: Meat, fish, dairy products, and fortified cereals.

o **Supplementation**: Available as cyanocobalamin or methylcobalamin in tablets or capsules.

Minerals

1. **Selenium**:
    o **Benefits**: Acts as an antioxidant, supports heart health, and reduces inflammation.
    o **Sources**: Brazil nuts, seafood, eggs, and whole grains.
    o **Supplementation**: Available as selenomethionine or sodium selenite in tablets or capsules.
2. **Zinc**:
    o **Benefits**: Supports immune function, reduces inflammation, and aids in tissue repair.
    o **Sources**: Meat, shellfish, legumes, and seeds.
    o **Supplementation**: Available as zinc gluconate or zinc citrate in tablets or capsules.
3. **Copper**:
    o **Benefits**: Essential for collagen formation, supports blood vessel health, and acts as an antioxidant.

- ○ **Sources**: Shellfish, nuts, seeds, and whole grains.
- ○ **Supplementation**: Available as copper gluconate or copper sulfate in tablets or capsules.

Supplements

1. **Nattokinase**:
   - ○ **Benefits**: An enzyme that helps dissolve blood clots, improving circulation and supporting heart health.
   - ○ **Sources**: Derived from natto, a fermented soybean product.
   - ○ **Supplementation**: Available in capsule form.
2. **Quercetin**:
   - ○ **Benefits**: A flavonoid with antioxidant and anti-inflammatory properties that support cardiovascular health.
   - ○ **Sources**: Onions, apples, berries, and tea.
   - ○ **Supplementation**: Available in tablet or capsule form.
3. **Resveratrol**:
   - ○ **Benefits**: Found in red wine and grapes, it has antioxidant

properties that support heart health and reduce inflammation.

- o **Sources**: Grapes, red wine, and berries.
- o **Supplementation**: Available in capsules or tablets.

4. **L-Arginine**:
   - o **Benefits**: An amino acid that helps produce nitric oxide, improving blood flow and supporting cardiovascular health.
   - o **Sources**: Meat, dairy, and legumes.
   - o **Supplementation**: Available in powder or capsule form

Pulmonary Valve

The pulmonary valve is one of the four main valves of the heart, playing a critical role in regulating blood flow from the right ventricle into the pulmonary artery. This valve ensures that deoxygenated blood is directed towards the lungs for oxygenation.

1. **Location**:
    - The pulmonary valve is situated between the right ventricle and the pulmonary artery.
2. **Anatomical Features**:
    - **Cusps**: The pulmonary valve consists of three semilunar cusps (anterior, right, and left) that open and close to regulate blood flow.
    - **Annulus**: A fibrous ring that provides structural support to the valve and anchors the cusps.
    - **Sinuses**: Small spaces behind the cusps that fill with blood to help close the valve.
3. **Function**:
    - During right ventricular systole, the pulmonary valve opens, allowing blood to flow from the right ventricle into the pulmonary

artery. During diastole, the valve closes to prevent backflow of blood into the right ventricle.

Function

1. **Blood Flow Regulation**:
   - The pulmonary valve ensures unidirectional blood flow from the right ventricle to the pulmonary artery, facilitating efficient pulmonary circulation.
2. **Prevention of Backflow**:
   - By closing during diastole, the pulmonary valve prevents the backflow of blood into the right ventricle, maintaining proper pressure and volume in the heart chambers.
3. **Synchronization with Heartbeat**:
   - The pulmonary valve opens and closes in coordination with the heart's electrical impulses, ensuring synchronized and efficient pumping action.

Blood Supply

1. **Arterial Supply**:
   - The pulmonary valve receives blood supply from the right

coronary artery, which provides oxygenated blood to the valve tissue and surrounding structures.

2. **Venous Drainage**:
    - Deoxygenated blood from the pulmonary valve area drains into the right atrium via small cardiac veins.

Pathophysiology

1. **Pulmonary Valve Stenosis**:
    - Narrowing of the pulmonary valve opening, restricting blood flow from the right ventricle to the pulmonary artery, leading to increased ventricular pressure and reduced oxygenation.
2. **Pulmonary Valve Regurgitation**:
    - A condition where the valve does not close properly, allowing blood to flow back into the right ventricle, causing volume overload and right ventricular hypertrophy.
3. **Congenital Defects**:
    - Conditions like Tetralogy of Fallot, where the pulmonary valve is malformed, leading to

improper function and potential cyanosis and heart failure.

4. **Infective Endocarditis**:
   - An infection of the pulmonary valve, often seen in patients with congenital heart defects or intravenous drug users, which can cause valve damage and lead to regurgitation or stenosis.

The pulmonary valve plays a vital role in pulmonary circulation, ensuring that deoxygenated blood is efficiently pumped to the lungs for oxygenation. Understanding its structure, function, and associated pathologies is crucial for diagnosing and managing conditions that affect this valve.

Herbs, Vitamins, Minerals, and Supplements for Pulmonary Valve Health

Supporting the health of the pulmonary valve is essential for maintaining optimal cardiovascular function. Here are some herbs, vitamins, minerals, and supplements that can help support, maintain, and heal the pulmonary valve.

Herbs

1. **Astragalus**:
    - **Benefits**: Supports heart health, enhances immune function, and reduces inflammation.
    - **Usage**: Available as a tea, tincture, or in capsule form.
2. **Bilberry**:
    - **Benefits**: Improves circulation, reduces inflammation, and supports vascular health.
    - **Usage**: Consumed as a tea, extract, or in capsule form.
3. **Hibiscus**:
    - **Benefits**: Contains antioxidants, supports heart health, and reduces blood pressure.
    - **Usage**: Commonly consumed as a tea or in extract form.
4. **Oregano**:
    - **Benefits**: Has anti-inflammatory properties, supports immune function, and improves cardiovascular health.
    - **Usage**: Used as a culinary herb, in tinctures, or in capsule form.

Vitamins

1. **Vitamin A:**
   - **Benefits**: Supports immune function, reduces inflammation, and helps maintain healthy tissues.
   - **Sources**: Carrots, sweet potatoes, spinach, and liver.
   - **Supplementation**: Available as retinyl palmitate or beta-carotene in tablets or capsules.
2. **Vitamin C:**
   - **Benefits**: Acts as an antioxidant, supports collagen formation, and reduces oxidative stress.
   - **Sources**: Citrus fruits, strawberries, bell peppers, and broccoli.
   - **Supplementation**: Available as ascorbic acid in tablets or capsules.
3. **Vitamin B3 (Niacin):**
   - **Benefits**: Supports cardiovascular health, reduces cholesterol levels, and improves blood flow.
   - **Sources**: Meat, fish, nuts, and green vegetables.

o **Supplementation**: Available as niacinamide or nicotinic acid in tablets or capsules.

Minerals

1. **Magnesium**:
   - o **Benefits**: Regulates heart rhythm, supports muscle function, and reduces blood pressure.
   - o **Sources**: Nuts, seeds, whole grains, and leafy green vegetables.
   - o **Supplementation**: Available as magnesium citrate, oxide, or glycinate.
2. **Calcium**:
   - o **Benefits**: Essential for heart muscle contraction, supports vascular health, and maintains proper cardiac function.
   - o **Sources**: Dairy products, fortified plant milks, and leafy green vegetables.
   - o **Supplementation**: Available as calcium carbonate or citrate.
3. **Phosphorus**:
   - o **Benefits**: Supports energy production in heart cells, helps

maintain healthy bones and teeth, and aids in muscle function.
  - **Sources**: Meat, fish, dairy products, and nuts.
  - **Supplementation**: Available as phosphate salts in tablets or capsules.

Supplements

1. **Coenzyme Q10 (CoQ10):**
   - **Benefits**: Supports energy production in heart cells, reduces oxidative stress, and improves overall heart function.
   - **Sources**: Meat, fish, and whole grains.
   - **Supplementation**: Available in capsule or tablet form.
2. **Taurine:**
   - **Benefits**: An amino acid that supports heart function, reduces blood pressure, and improves circulation.
   - **Sources**: Meat, fish, and dairy products.
   - **Supplementation**: Available in powder or capsule form.
3. **L-Carnitine:**

- **Benefits**: Supports energy production in heart cells, enhances fat metabolism, and improves cardiovascular health.
  - **Sources**: Meat, fish, and dairy products.
  - **Supplementation**: Available in liquid, capsule, or tablet form.
4. **Omega-3 Fatty Acids**:
  - **Benefits**: Found in fish oil and flaxseed, they reduce inflammation, support heart health, and improve vascular function.
  - **Sources**: Fatty fish, flaxseeds, and walnuts.
  - **Supplementation**: Available in capsule or liquid form.

Mitral Valve

The mitral valve, also known as the bicuspid valve, is one of the four main valves in the heart. It plays a critical role in regulating blood flow between the left atrium and the left ventricle, ensuring that oxygenated blood flows efficiently from the lungs to the rest of the body.

1. **Location**:
    - The mitral valve is located between the left atrium and the left ventricle.
2. **Anatomical Features**:
    - **Leaflets**: The mitral valve consists of two cusps or leaflets—anterior and posterior—that open and close to regulate blood flow.
    - **Chordae Tendineae**: Tendinous cords connecting the leaflets to the papillary muscles, preventing the leaflets from prolapsing into the atrium during ventricular contraction.
    - **Papillary Muscles**: Small muscles within the left ventricle that anchor the chordae

tendineae and aid in valve function.

- **Annulus**: A fibrous ring that provides structural support to the valve and anchors the leaflets.

3. **Function**:
   - During atrial systole, the mitral valve opens, allowing blood to flow from the left atrium to the left ventricle. During ventricular systole, the valve closes to prevent backflow of blood into the left atrium.

Function

1. **Blood Flow Regulation**:
   - The mitral valve ensures unidirectional blood flow from the left atrium to the left ventricle, facilitating efficient systemic circulation.

2. **Prevention of Backflow**:
   - By closing during ventricular contraction, the mitral valve prevents the backflow of blood into the left atrium, maintaining proper pressure and volume in the heart chambers.

3. **Synchronization with Heartbeat**:

- o The mitral valve opens and closes in coordination with the heart's electrical impulses, ensuring synchronized and efficient pumping action.

Blood Supply

1. **Arterial Supply**:
   - o The mitral valve is supplied by branches of the left coronary artery, which provides oxygenated blood to the valve tissue and surrounding structures.
2. **Venous Drainage**:
   - o Deoxygenated blood from the mitral valve area drains into the coronary sinus and then into the right atrium.

Pathophysiology

1. **Mitral Valve Prolapse**:
   - o A condition where the valve leaflets bulge into the left atrium during ventricular contraction, potentially causing regurgitation.
2. **Mitral Valve Regurgitation**:

- Occurs when the valve does not close properly, allowing blood to flow back into the left atrium, leading to symptoms like fatigue, shortness of breath, and arrhythmias.

3. **Mitral Valve Stenosis**:
   - Narrowing of the mitral valve opening, restricting blood flow from the left atrium to the left ventricle, causing increased atrial pressure and pulmonary congestion.

4. **Infective Endocarditis**:
   - An infection of the mitral valve, which can cause valve damage and lead to regurgitation or stenosis.

The mitral valve is essential for the proper functioning of the heart, ensuring that oxygenated blood flows efficiently from the left atrium to the left ventricle and preventing backflow. Understanding its structure, function, and associated pathologies is crucial for diagnosing and managing conditions that affect this valve.

Herbs, Vitamins, Minerals, and Supplements for Mitral Valve Health

Maintaining the health of the mitral valve is vital for overall cardiovascular function. Here are some herbs, vitamins, minerals, and supplements that can help support, maintain, and heal the mitral valve.

Herbs

1. **Hawthorn**:
    - **Benefits**: Strengthens heart muscle, improves blood flow, and supports overall cardiovascular health.
    - **Usage**: Available as a tea, tincture, or in capsule form.
2. **Motherwort**:
    - **Benefits**: Supports heart health, reduces palpitations, and has calming effects on the nervous system.
    - **Usage**: Consumed as a tea, extract, or in capsule form.
3. **Olive Leaf**:
    - **Benefits**: Contains antioxidants, supports heart health, and reduces inflammation.

- **Usage**: Commonly consumed as a tea or in extract form.

4. **Dandelion**:
   - **Benefits**: Acts as a diuretic, reduces blood pressure, and supports cardiovascular health.
   - **Usage**: Used as a tea, in tinctures, or in capsule form.

Vitamins

1. **Vitamin E**:
   - **Benefits**: Acts as an antioxidant, supports cardiovascular health, and reduces oxidative stress.
   - **Sources**: Nuts, seeds, spinach, and broccoli.
   - **Supplementation**: Available as tocopherol or tocotrienol in tablets or capsules.
2. **Vitamin B6 (Pyridoxine)**:
   - **Benefits**: Supports red blood cell production, reduces homocysteine levels, and improves heart health.
   - **Sources**: Poultry, fish, potatoes, and non-citrus fruits.
   - **Supplementation**: Available as pyridoxine hydrochloride in tablets or capsules.

3. **Vitamin B9 (Folic Acid)**:
    - **Benefits**: Reduces homocysteine levels, supports heart health, and aids in red blood cell formation.
    - **Sources**: Leafy green vegetables, legumes, and fortified cereals.
    - **Supplementation**: Available as folic acid in tablets or capsules.

Minerals

1. **Potassium**:
    - **Benefits**: Regulates heart rhythm, supports muscle function, and helps maintain proper cardiac function.
    - **Sources**: Bananas, oranges, potatoes, and spinach.
    - **Supplementation**: Available as potassium chloride or potassium gluconate in tablets or capsules.
2. **Sodium**:
    - **Benefits**: Essential for nerve function, helps regulate blood pressure, and maintains fluid balance.
    - **Sources**: Salt, processed foods, and natural sources like vegetables.

- ○ **Supplementation**: Generally obtained through diet, but available in electrolyte supplements.
3. **Chloride**:
    - ○ **Benefits**: Helps maintain fluid balance, supports nerve function, and aids in digestion.
    - ○ **Sources**: Salt, seaweed, rye, and tomatoes.
    - ○ **Supplementation**: Generally obtained through diet, but available in electrolyte supplements.

Supplements

1. **L-Arginine**:
    - ○ **Benefits**: An amino acid that helps produce nitric oxide, improving blood flow and supporting cardiovascular health.
    - ○ **Sources**: Meat, dairy, and legumes.
    - ○ **Supplementation**: Available in powder or capsule form.
2. **L-Citrulline**:
    - ○ **Benefits**: An amino acid that supports nitric oxide production,

improves circulation, and enhances cardiovascular health.

- o **Sources**: Watermelon, cucumbers, and gourds.
- o **Supplementation**: Available in powder or capsule form.

3. **Alpha-Lipoic Acid**:
   - o **Benefits**: Acts as an antioxidant, supports heart health, and reduces oxidative stress.
   - o **Sources**: Spinach, broccoli, and organ meats.
   - o **Supplementation**: Available in tablet or capsule form.

4. **Magnesium Taurate**:
   - o **Benefits**: Combines magnesium and taurine to support heart function, reduce blood pressure, and improve cardiovascular health.
   - o **Sources**: Not typically found in foods, primarily available as a supplement.
   - o **Supplementation**: Available in capsule or tablet form.

Aortic Valve

The aortic valve is one of the four main valves in the heart. It plays a crucial role in regulating blood flow from the left ventricle into the aorta and ensuring that oxygenated blood is efficiently distributed to the body.

1. **Location**:
    - The aortic valve is located between the left ventricle and the aorta, the largest artery in the body.
2. **Anatomical Features**:
    - **Cusps**: The aortic valve consists of three semilunar cusps (right coronary cusp, left coronary cusp, and non-coronary cusp) that open and close to regulate blood flow.
    - **Annulus**: A fibrous ring that provides structural support to the valve and anchors the cusps.
    - **Sinuses of Valsalva**: These are the spaces just above the cusps where the aorta begins, and they help in the closure of the valve.
3. **Function**:

- During left ventricular systole, the aortic valve opens, allowing blood to flow from the left ventricle into the aorta. During diastole, the valve closes to prevent backflow of blood into the left ventricle.

Function

1. **Blood Flow Regulation**:
   - The aortic valve ensures unidirectional blood flow from the left ventricle to the aorta, facilitating efficient systemic circulation.
2. **Prevention of Backflow**:
   - By closing during ventricular relaxation (diastole), the aortic valve prevents the backflow of blood into the left ventricle, maintaining proper pressure and volume in the heart chambers.
3. **Synchronization with Heartbeat**:
   - The aortic valve opens and closes in coordination with the heart's electrical impulses, ensuring synchronized and efficient pumping action.

Blood Supply

1. **Arterial Supply**:
   - The aortic valve receives blood supply from the coronary arteries, which arise from the right and left coronary cusps.
2. **Venous Drainage**:
   - Deoxygenated blood from the aortic valve area drains into the coronary sinus and then into the right atrium.

Pathophysiology

1. **Aortic Stenosis**:
   - Narrowing of the aortic valve opening, restricting blood flow from the left ventricle to the aorta, leading to increased ventricular pressure and hypertrophy.
2. **Aortic Regurgitation**:
   - A condition where the valve does not close properly, allowing blood to flow back into the left ventricle, causing volume overload and left ventricular dilation.
3. **Congenital Defects**:

- Conditions like bicuspid aortic valve, where the valve has two cusps instead of three, leading to abnormal function and potential complications like stenosis or regurgitation.
4. **Infective Endocarditis**:
    - An infection of the aortic valve, which can cause valve damage and lead to regurgitation or stenosis.

The aortic valve is essential for the proper functioning of the heart, ensuring that oxygenated blood flows efficiently from the left ventricle into the aorta and preventing backflow. Understanding its structure, function, and associated pathologies is crucial for diagnosing and managing conditions that affect this valve.

Herbs, Vitamins, Minerals, and Supplements for Aortic Valve Health

Maintaining the health of the aortic valve is vital for overall cardiovascular function. Here are some herbs, vitamins, minerals, and supplements that can help support, maintain, and heal the aortic valve.

Herbs

1. **Ginkgo Biloba**:
   - **Benefits**: Enhances circulation, reduces inflammation, and supports overall cardiovascular health.
   - **Usage**: Available as a tea, extract, or in capsule form.
2. **Cayenne Pepper**:
   - **Benefits**: Improves blood flow, supports heart health, and reduces blood pressure.
   - **Usage**: Consumed as a spice, in tinctures, or in capsule form.
3. **Garlic**:
   - **Benefits**: Reduces cholesterol levels, supports cardiovascular health, and has anti-inflammatory properties.

- o **Usage**: Consumed raw, cooked, or as a supplement in capsule form.

4. **Turmeric**:
   - o **Benefits**: Contains curcumin, which has anti-inflammatory and antioxidant properties, supporting heart health.
   - o **Usage**: Used as a spice, in teas, or in supplement form.

Vitamins

1. **Vitamin K2**:
   - o **Benefits**: Supports calcium regulation in the arteries, preventing calcification and supporting vascular health.
   - o **Sources**: Fermented foods, dairy products, and leafy greens.
   - o **Supplementation**: Available as menaquinone-7 (MK-7) in tablets or capsules.

2. **Vitamin D3**:
   - o **Benefits**: Supports heart health, enhances calcium absorption, and reduces inflammation.
   - o **Sources**: Sunlight, fatty fish, and fortified foods.

- **Supplementation**: Available as cholecalciferol in tablets or capsules.

3. **Vitamin B12 (Cobalamin)**:
   - **Benefits**: Supports red blood cell production, reduces homocysteine levels, and improves heart health.
   - **Sources**: Meat, fish, dairy, and fortified cereals.
   - **Supplementation**: Available as cyanocobalamin or methylcobalamin in tablets or capsules.

Minerals

1. **Zinc**:
   - **Benefits**: Supports immune function, reduces inflammation, and aids in tissue repair.
   - **Sources**: Meat, shellfish, legumes, and seeds.
   - **Supplementation**: Available as zinc gluconate or zinc sulfate in tablets or capsules.

2. **Selenium**:
   - **Benefits**: Acts as an antioxidant, supports heart health, and reduces oxidative stress.

- ○ **Sources**: Brazil nuts, fish, and eggs.
  - ○ **Supplementation**: Available as selenomethionine in tablets or capsules.

3. **Copper**:
   - ○ **Benefits**: Supports heart health, enhances iron absorption, and aids in the formation of red blood cells.
   - ○ **Sources**: Shellfish, nuts, seeds, and whole grains.
   - ○ **Supplementation**: Available as copper gluconate or copper sulfate in tablets or capsules.

Supplements

1. **Resveratrol**:
   - ○ **Benefits**: Found in red wine and grapes, it supports heart health, reduces inflammation, and acts as an antioxidant.
   - ○ **Sources**: Red grapes, berries, and red wine.
   - ○ **Supplementation**: Available in tablet or capsule form.
2. **Pomegranate Extract**:

- **Benefits**: Contains antioxidants, supports heart health, and reduces arterial plaque.
  - **Sources**: Pomegranate fruit.
  - **Supplementation**: Available in juice, tablet, or capsule form.
3. **Green Tea Extract**:
  - **Benefits**: Contains catechins, supports heart health, and reduces blood pressure.
  - **Sources**: Green tea.
  - **Supplementation**: Available in tablet or capsule form.
4. **Nattokinase**:
  - **Benefits**: An enzyme derived from natto (fermented soybeans) that supports cardiovascular health and reduces blood clotting.
  - **Sources**: Natto.
  - **Supplementation**: Available in capsule form.

Pulmonary Circulation

Pulmonary circulation is the portion of the cardiovascular system that carries deoxygenated blood away from the right side of the heart, to the lungs, and returns oxygenated blood to the left side of the heart. This process is crucial for gas exchange, enabling the blood to release carbon dioxide and absorb oxygen.

Components and Pathway

1. **Right Atrium**:
    - **Function**: Receives deoxygenated blood from the body via the superior and inferior vena cava.
    - **Pathway**: Blood flows from the right atrium through the tricuspid valve into the right ventricle.
2. **Right Ventricle**:
    - **Function**: Pumps deoxygenated blood into the pulmonary circulation.
    - **Pathway**: Blood flows from the right ventricle through the pulmonary valve into the pulmonary artery.
3. **Pulmonary Artery**:

- **Structure**: Divides into the left
    and right pulmonary arteries,
    which carry blood to the
    respective lungs.
  - **Function**: Transports
    deoxygenated blood from the
    right ventricle to the lungs.
4. **Lungs**:
  - **Function**: Site of gas exchange
    where blood releases carbon
    dioxide and picks up oxygen.
  - **Components**: Alveoli (air sacs)
    where the actual gas exchange
    occurs.
5. **Pulmonary Veins**:
  - **Structure**: Four veins (two from
    each lung) that carry oxygenated
    blood.
  - **Function**: Transport oxygenated
    blood from the lungs to the left
    atrium.
6. **Left Atrium**:
  - **Function**: Receives oxygenated
    blood from the pulmonary veins.
  - **Pathway**: Blood flows from the
    left atrium through the mitral
    valve into the left ventricle.
7. **Left Ventricle**:

- **Function**: Pumps oxygenated blood into the systemic circulation to supply the body.
  - **Pathway**: Blood flows from the left ventricle through the aortic valve into the aorta and systemic circulation.

Gas Exchange Process

1. **Inhalation**:
   - Oxygen enters the lungs through the bronchi and reaches the alveoli.
2. **Diffusion**:
   - Oxygen diffuses across the thin walls of the alveoli into the capillaries.
   - Carbon dioxide diffuses from the blood into the alveoli to be exhaled.
3. **Exhalation**:
   - Carbon dioxide is expelled from the lungs during exhalation.
4. **Oxygen Transport**:
   - Oxygen binds to hemoglobin in red blood cells, which then transport it to the heart via pulmonary veins.

Regulation

1. **Autonomic Nervous System**:
    - Controls the rate and depth of breathing, adjusting pulmonary circulation based on the body's oxygen needs.
2. **Chemoreceptors**:
    - Located in the carotid and aortic bodies, they detect changes in blood pH, CO_2, and O_2 levels, signaling the respiratory centers in the brain to adjust breathing.
3. **Pulmonary Blood Flow**:
    - Regulated to match ventilation with perfusion (V/Q ratio), ensuring efficient gas exchange.

Pathophysiology

1. **Pulmonary Hypertension**:
    - Increased blood pressure within the pulmonary arteries, leading to right ventricular hypertrophy and heart failure if untreated.
2. **Pulmonary Embolism**:
    - Blockage of a pulmonary artery by a blood clot, fat, or air bubble, which can impair blood flow and gas exchange.

3. **Chronic Obstructive Pulmonary Disease (COPD)**:
   - Includes conditions like emphysema and chronic bronchitis, leading to obstructed airflow and impaired gas exchange.
4. **Acute Respiratory Distress Syndrome (ARDS)**:
   - Severe inflammation and fluid buildup in the alveoli, leading to impaired oxygen exchange and respiratory failure.

Pulmonary circulation is an essential component of the cardiovascular system, enabling gas exchange that oxygenates blood and removes carbon dioxide. Understanding its structure, function, and regulation is crucial for diagnosing and managing various cardiovascular and respiratory conditions.

Herbs, Vitamins, Minerals, and Supplements for Pulmonary Circulation Health

Supporting pulmonary circulation involves maintaining heart and lung health, enhancing oxygenation, and reducing inflammation. Here are some herbs, vitamins, minerals, and supplements that can help support, maintain, and heal the pulmonary circulation.

Herbs

1. **Mullein**:
    - **Benefits**: Supports respiratory health, reduces inflammation, and aids in clearing mucus.
    - **Usage**: Available as a tea, tincture, or in capsule form.
2. **Lobelia**:
    - **Benefits**: Acts as a bronchodilator, easing breathing and supporting lung function.
    - **Usage**: Consumed as a tea, in tinctures, or in capsule form.
3. **Elecampane**:
    - **Benefits**: Supports respiratory health, has expectorant properties, and reduces inflammation.

- ○ **Usage**: Used as a tea, in tinctures, or in capsule form.
4. **Thyme**:
   - ○ **Benefits**: Contains thymol, which has antimicrobial properties and supports respiratory health.
   - ○ **Usage**: Used as a spice, in teas, or in extract form.

Vitamins

1. **Vitamin C**:
   - ○ **Benefits**: Supports immune function, reduces inflammation, and aids in collagen formation for healthy blood vessels.
   - ○ **Sources**: Citrus fruits, strawberries, bell peppers, and broccoli.
   - ○ **Supplementation**: Available as ascorbic acid in tablets or capsules.
2. **Vitamin A**:
   - ○ **Benefits**: Supports respiratory health, enhances immune function, and maintains mucosal surfaces.

- **Sources**: Carrots, sweet potatoes, spinach, and fish liver oil.
  - **Supplementation**: Available as retinol or beta-carotene in tablets or capsules.
3. **Vitamin E**:
  - **Benefits**: Acts as an antioxidant, supports cardiovascular health, and reduces oxidative stress.
  - **Sources**: Nuts, seeds, spinach, and broccoli.
  - **Supplementation**: Available as tocopherol in tablets or capsules.

Minerals

1. **Magnesium**:
  - **Benefits**: Supports muscle relaxation, including bronchial muscles, and reduces inflammation.
  - **Sources**: Nuts, seeds, whole grains, and leafy greens.
  - **Supplementation**: Available as magnesium citrate or magnesium glycinate in tablets or capsules.
2. **Calcium**:
  - **Benefits**: Supports cardiovascular health, aids in

muscle function, and maintains healthy blood vessels.

- ○ **Sources**: Dairy products, leafy greens, and fortified foods.
- ○ **Supplementation**: Available as calcium carbonate or calcium citrate in tablets or capsules.

3. **Iron**:
- ○ **Benefits**: Essential for hemoglobin formation, which is crucial for oxygen transport in the blood.
- ○ **Sources**: Red meat, beans, lentils, and fortified cereals.
- ○ **Supplementation**: Available as ferrous sulfate or ferrous gluconate in tablets or capsules.

Supplements

1. **Omega-3 Fatty Acids**:
- ○ **Benefits**: Support cardiovascular health, reduce inflammation, and improve endothelial function.
- ○ **Sources**: Fatty fish, flaxseeds, and chia seeds.
- ○ **Supplementation**: Available as fish oil or flaxseed oil in capsules.

2. **Coenzyme Q10 (CoQ10)**:

- **Benefits**: Supports heart health, improves energy production in cells, and acts as an antioxidant.
  - **Sources**: Meat, fish, and whole grains.
  - **Supplementation**: Available in tablet or capsule form.
3. **N-Acetylcysteine (NAC)**:
  - **Benefits**: Acts as a precursor to glutathione, supports lung health, and reduces mucus production.
  - **Sources**: Naturally occurring in certain foods, but primarily available as a supplement.
  - **Supplementation**: Available in tablet or capsule form.
4. **Quercetin**:
  - **Benefits**: Acts as an antioxidant, supports respiratory health, and reduces inflammation.
  - **Sources**: Onions, apples, and berries.
  - **Supplementation**: Available in tablet or capsule form.

Systemic Circulation

Systemic circulation is the part of the cardiovascular system responsible for carrying oxygenated blood from the heart to the body and returning deoxygenated blood back to the heart. This process ensures that all body tissues receive the oxygen and nutrients they need for proper function and removes carbon dioxide and metabolic waste products.

Components and Pathway

1. **Left Ventricle**:
    - **Function**: Pumps oxygenated blood into the systemic circulation.
    - **Pathway**: Blood flows from the left ventricle through the aortic valve into the aorta.
2. **Aorta**:
    - **Structure**: The largest artery in the body, branching into major arteries that supply different body regions.
    - **Function**: Distributes oxygenated blood to all systemic arteries.
3. **Arteries and Arterioles**:

- **Function**: Carry oxygen-rich blood away from the heart to the tissues.
    - **Structure**: Arteries branch into smaller arterioles which lead to capillaries.
4. **Capillaries**:
    - **Function**: Site of nutrient, gas, and waste exchange between blood and tissues.
    - **Structure**: Thin-walled vessels that allow for efficient exchange at the cellular level.
5. **Veins and Venules**:
    - **Function**: Carry deoxygenated blood back to the heart.
    - **Structure**: Capillaries merge into venules, which then form veins.
6. **Superior and Inferior Vena Cava**:
    - **Function**: Large veins that return deoxygenated blood to the right atrium of the heart.
    - **Pathway**: Blood from the upper body drains into the superior vena cava, while blood from the lower body drains into the inferior vena cava.
7. **Right Atrium**:

- **Function**: Receives deoxygenated blood from the systemic veins.
- **Pathway**: Blood flows from the right atrium through the tricuspid valve into the right ventricle, where it will be sent to the pulmonary circulation for oxygenation.

Regulation

1. **Autonomic Nervous System**:
   - **Sympathetic Nervous System**: Increases heart rate and contractility, constricts blood vessels to increase blood pressure.
   - **Parasympathetic Nervous System**: Decreases heart rate and dilates blood vessels to lower blood pressure.
2. **Hormonal Control**:
   - **Epinephrine and Norepinephrine**: Increase heart rate and contractility, constrict blood vessels.
   - **Renin-Angiotensin-Aldosterone System (RAAS)**: Regulates blood pressure and fluid balance

by controlling blood vessel
constriction and sodium
retention.

3. **Local Control**:
   - **Autoregulation**: Tissues
     regulate their own blood flow by
     altering the diameter of arterioles
     in response to local factors such
     as oxygen and carbon dioxide
     levels.

Pathophysiology

1. **Hypertension**:
   - Chronic high blood pressure that
     can lead to damage of the blood
     vessels and organs.
   - Increases the risk of heart
     disease, stroke, and kidney
     failure.
2. **Atherosclerosis**:
   - Buildup of plaques in the arteries,
     leading to narrowed and stiffened
     arteries.
   - Can result in reduced blood flow,
     heart attacks, and strokes.
3. **Heart Failure**:
   - The heart's inability to pump
     blood effectively, leading to

inadequate blood flow to meet the body's needs.

- ○ Symptoms include shortness of breath, fatigue, and fluid retention.

4. **Peripheral Artery Disease (PAD)**:
   - ○ Narrowing of the arteries in the limbs, often causing pain and limited mobility.
   - ○ Increases the risk of infection and limb amputation.

Herbs, Vitamins, Minerals, and Supplements for Systemic Circulation Health

Maintaining the health of systemic circulation involves supporting cardiovascular health, enhancing blood flow, and reducing inflammation. Here are some herbs, vitamins, minerals, and supplements that can help support, maintain, and heal the systemic circulation.

Herbs

1. **Hawthorn:**

- **Benefits**: Supports heart health, improves blood flow, and strengthens blood vessels.
  - **Usage**: Available as tea, tincture, or in capsule form.
2. **Ginkgo Biloba**:
  - **Benefits**: Enhances blood flow, especially to the extremities and brain, and has antioxidant properties.
  - **Usage**: Available as a tea, extract, or in capsule form.
3. **Garlic**:
  - **Benefits**: Reduces blood pressure, lowers cholesterol levels, and improves blood circulation.
  - **Usage**: Consumed fresh, as a supplement, or in extract form.
4. **Cayenne Pepper**:
  - **Benefits**: Improves circulation, strengthens the cardiovascular system, and has anti-inflammatory properties.
  - **Usage**: Used as a spice, in teas, or in capsule form.

Vitamins

1. **Vitamin K**:

- o **Benefits**: Supports blood clotting and maintains healthy blood vessels.
    - o **Sources**: Leafy green vegetables, broccoli, and Brussels sprouts.
    - o **Supplementation**: Available in tablets or capsules.
2. **Vitamin B6 (Pyridoxine)**:
    - o **Benefits**: Supports red blood cell production and maintains healthy blood vessels.
    - o **Sources**: Poultry, fish, potatoes, and bananas.
    - o **Supplementation**: Available in tablets or capsules.
3. **Vitamin B12 (Cobalamin)**:
    - o **Benefits**: Supports red blood cell production and maintains nerve health.
    - o **Sources**: Meat, dairy products, and fortified cereals.
    - o **Supplementation**: Available in tablets or capsules.

Minerals

1. **Potassium**:
    - o **Benefits**: Maintains proper heart function and regulates blood pressure.

- o **Sources**: Bananas, oranges, potatoes, and spinach.
- o **Supplementation**: Available in tablets or capsules.

2. **Zinc**:
   - o **Benefits**: Supports immune function and maintains the health of blood vessels.
   - o **Sources**: Meat, shellfish, legumes, and seeds.
   - o **Supplementation**: Available in tablets or capsules.

3. **Selenium**:
   - o **Benefits**: Acts as an antioxidant, supports cardiovascular health, and reduces inflammation.
   - o **Sources**: Brazil nuts, seafood, and eggs.
   - o **Supplementation**: Available in tablets or capsules.

Supplements

1. **L-Arginine**:
   - o **Benefits**: An amino acid that improves blood flow and supports cardiovascular health by producing nitric oxide.
   - o **Sources**: Meat, dairy, and nuts.

- **Supplementation**: Available in powder or capsule form.

2. **Taurine**:
   - **Benefits**: An amino acid that supports cardiovascular health, improves blood flow, and reduces oxidative stress.
   - **Sources**: Meat, fish, and dairy products.
   - **Supplementation**: Available in powder or capsule form.

3. **Resveratrol**:
   - **Benefits**: An antioxidant found in red wine and grapes that supports cardiovascular health and reduces inflammation.
   - **Sources**: Grapes, red wine, and berries.
   - **Supplementation**: Available in tablet or capsule form.

4. **Pycnogenol (Pine Bark Extract)**:
   - **Benefits**: Improves blood flow, reduces blood pressure, and has antioxidant properties.
   - **Sources**: Extracted from the bark of the French maritime pine tree.
   - **Supplementation**: Available in tablet or capsule form

Electrical Conduction System of the Heart

The electrical conduction system of the heart is essential for coordinating the heart's rhythm and ensuring efficient pumping of blood. This system generates and transmits electrical impulses that stimulate the heart muscle to contract in a synchronized manner. Here's a detailed breakdown of its components and function:

Components of the Electrical Conduction System

1. **Sinoatrial (SA) Node:**
    - **Location**: Upper wall of the right atrium, near the opening of the superior vena cava.
    - **Function**: Acts as the heart's natural pacemaker by generating electrical impulses at regular intervals.
    - **Mechanism**: The impulses produced by the SA node cause the atria to contract, pushing blood into the ventricles.
2. **Atrioventricular (AV) Node:**

- **Location**: Lower part of the right atrium, near the interatrial septum.
- **Function**: Delays the electrical impulse from the atria before transmitting it to the ventricles, ensuring the atria have time to fully contract and the ventricles to fill with blood.
- **Mechanism**: This delay is crucial for maintaining the proper timing of the cardiac cycle.

3. **Bundle of His (Atrioventricular Bundle)**:
   - **Location**: Starts at the AV node and runs down the interventricular septum.
   - **Function**: Transmits the electrical impulse from the AV node to the ventricles.
   - **Mechanism**: The bundle of His splits into right and left bundle branches that extend into the ventricles.
4. **Right and Left Bundle Branches**:
   - **Location**: Extend from the bundle of His through the interventricular septum into the

walls of the right and left ventricles.

- o **Function**: Carry the electrical impulses to the Purkinje fibers in the ventricles.
- o **Mechanism**: These branches ensure that the impulses are distributed evenly across both ventricles for synchronized contraction.

5. **Purkinje Fibers**:
   - o **Location**: Network of fibers spread throughout the ventricles' inner walls.
   - o **Function**: Rapidly conduct the electrical impulses to the ventricular muscle cells.
   - o **Mechanism**: This causes the ventricles to contract, pumping blood out of the heart to the lungs and the rest of the body.

Sequence of Electrical Conduction

1. **Impulse Generation**:
   - o The SA node generates an electrical impulse.
   - o This impulse spreads across the walls of the atria, causing atrial contraction.

2. **Impulse Transmission to the AV Node**:
    - The electrical impulse reaches the AV node.
    - The AV node delays the impulse to allow the ventricles to fill with blood.
3. **Impulse Transmission to the Bundle of His**:
    - From the AV node, the impulse travels down the bundle of His.
    - The bundle of His divides into right and left bundle branches.
4. **Impulse Distribution via Purkinje Fibers**:
    - The right and left bundle branches transmit the impulse to the Purkinje fibers.
    - The Purkinje fibers distribute the impulse throughout the ventricular muscle cells.
5. **Ventricular Contraction**:
    - The impulse causes the ventricles to contract.
    - Blood is pumped from the right ventricle to the lungs and from the left ventricle to the rest of the body.

Regulation and Pathophysiology

1. **Autonomic Nervous System**:
    - **Sympathetic Nervous System**: Increases heart rate and force of contraction.
    - **Parasympathetic Nervous System**: Decreases heart rate.
2. **Electrolyte Balance**:
    - Proper levels of potassium, calcium, and sodium are crucial for the generation and conduction of electrical impulses.
3. **Arrhythmias**:
    - Abnormalities in the electrical conduction system can lead to arrhythmias, where the heart beats too fast, too slow, or irregularly.
    - Common types include atrial fibrillation, ventricular tachycardia, and heart block.
4. **Conduction Block**:
    - A blockage or delay in the electrical pathway, such as in bundle branch block, can disrupt the synchronized contraction of the heart.

Herbs, Vitamins, Minerals, and Supplements for Supporting the Electrical Conduction System

Maintaining a healthy electrical conduction system is crucial for overall heart health. Certain herbs, vitamins, minerals, and supplements can support heart function, enhance electrical conduction, and reduce the risk of arrhythmias.

Herbs

1. **Motherwort:**
   - **Benefits**: Supports heart rhythm and reduces palpitations.
   - **Usage**: Available as tea, tincture, or in capsule form.
2. **Lemon Balm:**
   - **Benefits**: Calms the nervous system and can help regulate heart rate.
   - **Usage**: Available as tea, extract, or in capsule form.
3. **Passionflower:**
   - **Benefits**: Reduces anxiety and can help stabilize heart rhythm.
   - **Usage**: Available as tea, tincture, or in capsule form.
4. **Reishi Mushroom:**

- Benefits: Supports
    cardiovascular health and has
    adaptogenic properties.
  - Usage: Available as a powder,
    extract, or in capsule form.

Vitamins

1. **Vitamin C:**
   - **Benefits**: Supports overall heart
     health and reduces oxidative
     stress.
   - **Sources**: Citrus fruits,
     strawberries, bell peppers.
   - **Supplementation**: Available in
     tablets or capsules.
2. **Vitamin D:**
   - **Benefits**: Maintains calcium
     balance, supporting proper heart
     function.
   - **Sources**: Sun exposure, fatty
     fish, fortified foods.
   - **Supplementation**: Available in
     tablets or capsules.
3. **Vitamin E:**
   - **Benefits**: Acts as an antioxidant
     and supports heart health.
   - **Sources**: Nuts, seeds, spinach.
   - **Supplementation**: Available in
     tablets or capsules.

Minerals

1. **Magnesium:**
   - **Benefits**: Supports heart rhythm and relaxes blood vessels.
   - **Sources**: Green leafy vegetables, nuts, seeds.
   - **Supplementation**: Available in tablets or capsules.
2. **Calcium:**
   - **Benefits**: Essential for muscle contraction and nerve function.
   - **Sources**: Dairy products, leafy green vegetables.
   - **Supplementation**: Available in tablets or capsules.
3. **Sodium:**
   - **Benefits**: Essential for nerve impulse transmission.
   - **Sources**: Table salt, processed foods.
   - **Supplementation**: Generally not needed unless there is a deficiency.

Supplements

1. **Coenzyme Q10 (CoQ10):**

- **Benefits**: Supports heart function and energy production in cells.
    - **Sources**: Found in small amounts in meat and fish.
    - **Supplementation**: Available in capsule or softgel form.
2. **Omega-3 Fatty Acids**:
    - **Benefits**: Reduce inflammation and support heart health.
    - **Sources**: Fatty fish, flaxseeds, walnuts.
    - **Supplementation**: Available in fish oil or flaxseed oil capsules.
3. **L-Carnitine**:
    - **Benefits**: Supports energy production in heart cells.
    - **Sources**: Found in small amounts in meat and dairy.
    - **Supplementation**: Available in capsule or liquid form.
4. **Taurine**:
    - **Benefits**: An amino acid that supports heart rhythm and reduces oxidative stress.
    - **Sources**: Found in meat, fish, and dairy.
    - **Supplementation**: Available in powder or capsule form.

Sinoatrial (SA) Node

The sinoatrial (SA) node, often referred to as the heart's natural pacemaker, is a critical component of the heart's electrical conduction system. It is responsible for initiating the electrical impulses that dictate the heart's rhythmic contractions.

1. **Location**:
    - The SA node is located in the right atrium of the heart, near the opening of the superior vena cava.
2. **Structure**:
    - The SA node is a small, specialized cluster of cardiac muscle cells.
    - These cells are unique in their ability to spontaneously generate electrical impulses.

Function

1. **Pacemaker Activity**:
    - The SA node generates electrical impulses at regular intervals, typically 60-100 times per minute in a healthy adult.

- ○ This automatic depolarization sets the pace for the entire heart, regulating its rhythm.
2. **Impulse Transmission**:
   - ○ The electrical impulses produced by the SA node spread through the walls of the atria, causing them to contract and push blood into the ventricles.
   - ○ These impulses then travel to the atrioventricular (AV) node, where they are delayed before being transmitted to the ventricles.

Mechanism of Action

1. **Generation of Electrical Impulses**:
   - ○ The SA node cells have a unique ability to depolarize spontaneously due to their high permeability to sodium and calcium ions.
   - ○ This depolarization creates an electrical impulse.
2. **Propagation of Impulses**:
   - ○ The generated impulse spreads rapidly through the atrial walls via gap junctions between cardiac cells.

- This coordinated spread of impulses ensures that the atria contract in unison.

3. **Atrial Contraction**:
   - The electrical impulse causes the atria to contract, pushing blood into the ventricles and priming the heart for the next phase of the cardiac cycle.

Regulation

1. **Autonomic Nervous System**:
   - **Sympathetic Nervous System**: Increases the rate of depolarization of the SA node, leading to an increased heart rate (positive chronotropic effect).
   - **Parasympathetic Nervous System (Vagus Nerve)**: Decreases the rate of depolarization of the SA node, leading to a decreased heart rate (negative chronotropic effect).
2. **Hormonal Influence**:
   - **Epinephrine and Norepinephrine**: Released by the adrenal glands, these hormones increase heart rate by stimulating the SA node.

- **Acetylcholine**: Released by the vagus nerve, this neurotransmitter decreases heart rate by inhibiting the SA node.

Pathophysiology

1. **Sinus Bradycardia**:
   - A condition where the SA node fires at a slower rate than normal, resulting in a slower heart rate.
   - Causes include increased vagal tone, hypothyroidism, and certain medications.
2. **Sinus Tachycardia**:
   - A condition where the SA node fires at a faster rate than normal, resulting in a faster heart rate.
   - Causes include fever, anxiety, hyperthyroidism, and certain stimulants.
3. **Sick Sinus Syndrome**:
   - A collection of heart rhythm disorders due to malfunction of the SA node.
   - Symptoms can include bradycardia, tachycardia, and irregular heart rhythms.

- o Treatment often involves medications or the implantation of a pacemaker.

Herbs, Vitamins, Minerals, and Supplements for Supporting SA Node Function

Maintaining the health and function of the SA node is crucial for overall heart rhythm and function. Several herbs, vitamins, minerals, and supplements can support the SA node's health and improve its function.

Herbs

1. **Motherwort (Leonurus cardiaca):**
   - o **Benefits**: Supports heart rhythm and reduces palpitations.
   - o **Usage**: Available as tea, tincture, or in capsule form.
2. **Lemon Balm (Melissa officinalis):**
   - o **Benefits**: Calms the nervous system and helps regulate heart rate.
   - o **Usage**: Available as tea, extract, or in capsule form.
3. **Hawthorn (Crataegus spp.):**

- **Benefits**: Strengthens the heart muscle and supports overall heart health.
    - **Usage**: Available as tea, tincture, or in capsule form.
4. **Passionflower (Passiflora incarnata)**:
    - **Benefits**: Reduces anxiety and can help stabilize heart rhythm.
    - **Usage**: Available as tea, tincture, or in capsule form.

Vitamins

1. **Vitamin B1 (Thiamine)**:
    - **Benefits**: Supports nerve function and heart health.
    - **Sources**: Whole grains, pork, legumes.
    - **Supplementation**: Available in tablets or capsules.
2. **Vitamin C (Ascorbic Acid)**:
    - **Benefits**: Supports overall cardiovascular health and reduces oxidative stress.
    - **Sources**: Citrus fruits, strawberries, bell peppers.
    - **Supplementation**: Available in tablets or capsules.
3. **Vitamin D**:

- o **Benefits**: Maintains calcium balance and supports proper heart function.
- o **Sources**: Sun exposure, fatty fish, fortified foods.
- o **Supplementation**: Available in tablets or capsules.

Minerals

1. **Magnesium**:
   - o **Benefits**: Supports heart rhythm and relaxes blood vessels.
   - o **Sources**: Green leafy vegetables, nuts, seeds.
   - o **Supplementation**: Available in tablets or capsules.
2. **Potassium**:
   - o **Benefits**: Essential for maintaining normal heart rhythm and muscle function.
   - o **Sources**: Bananas, oranges, potatoes, spinach.
   - o **Supplementation**: Available in tablets or capsules.
3. **Calcium**:
   - o **Benefits**: Necessary for muscle contraction and nerve function.
   - o **Sources**: Dairy products, leafy green vegetables.

- Supplementation: Available in tablets or capsules.

Supplements

1. **Coenzyme Q10 (CoQ10):**
   - **Benefits**: Supports heart function and energy production in cells.
   - **Sources**: Found in small amounts in meat and fish.
   - **Supplementation**: Available in capsule or softgel form.
2. **Omega-3 Fatty Acids**:
   - **Benefits**: Reduce inflammation and support heart health.
   - **Sources**: Fatty fish, flaxseeds, walnuts.
   - **Supplementation**: Available in fish oil or flaxseed oil capsules.
3. **L-Carnitine**:
   - **Benefits**: Supports energy production in heart cells.
   - **Sources**: Found in small amounts in meat and dairy.
   - **Supplementation**: Available in capsule or liquid form.
4. **Taurine:**

- **Benefits**: An amino acid that supports heart rhythm and reduces oxidative stress.
- **Sources**: Found in meat, fish, and dairy.
- **Supplementation**: Available in powder or capsule form

Atrioventricular (AV) Node

The atrioventricular (AV) node is a critical component of the heart's electrical conduction system. It acts as a gatekeeper for electrical impulses between the atria and the ventricles, ensuring that the heart beats in a coordinated and efficient manner.

1. **Location**:
   - The AV node is located in the lower part of the right atrium, near the interatrial septum and close to the tricuspid valve.
2. **Structure**:
   - The AV node is a small mass of specialized cardiac muscle cells.
   - These cells are interconnected and capable of transmitting electrical impulses.

Function

1. **Delay Conduction**:
   - The primary function of the AV node is to delay the transmission of electrical impulses from the atria to the ventricles.

- o   This delay allows the atria to complete their contraction and ensures that the ventricles have enough time to fill with blood before they contract.

2. **Secondary Pacemaker**:
    - o   The AV node can act as a secondary pacemaker if the SA node fails.
    - o   It generates impulses at a slower rate (40-60 beats per minute) compared to the SA node.

Mechanism of Action

1. **Impulse Reception from SA Node**:
    - o   Electrical impulses generated by the SA node travel through the atrial walls and reach the AV node.
    - o   The atria contract as these impulses pass through, pushing blood into the ventricles.

2. **Impulse Delay**:
    - o   The AV node slows down the electrical impulse to ensure a delay between atrial and ventricular contraction.
    - o   This delay is due to the smaller diameter of AV node cells and

fewer gap junctions, which slow impulse conduction.

3. **Impulse Transmission to the Bundle of His**:
    - After the delay, the AV node transmits the impulse to the bundle of His.
    - The bundle of His then conducts the impulse to the right and left bundle branches and eventually to the Purkinje fibers, causing the ventricles to contract.

Regulation

1. **Autonomic Nervous System:**
    - **Sympathetic Nervous System**: Increases the speed of impulse conduction through the AV node, leading to a shorter delay and a higher heart rate.
    - **Parasympathetic Nervous System (Vagus Nerve)**: Decreases the speed of impulse conduction, leading to a longer delay and a lower heart rate.
2. **Hormonal Influence**:
    - **Epinephrine and Norepinephrine**: These hormones increase the speed of

impulse conduction through the
AV node.

- o **Acetylcholine**: Released by the
  vagus nerve, it decreases the
  speed of impulse conduction
  through the AV node.

Pathophysiology

1. **AV Block**:
   - o A condition where the
     transmission of electrical
     impulses through the AV node is
     partially or completely blocked.
   - o Types of AV block include
     first-degree, second-degree
     (Mobitz type I and type II), and
     third-degree (complete) AV
     block.
2. **Junctional Rhythms**:
   - o If the SA node fails or the impulse
     is blocked, the AV node can take
     over as the primary pacemaker,
     leading to junctional rhythms.
   - o These rhythms are typically
     slower than those initiated by the
     SA node.
3. **AV Nodal Reentrant Tachycardia
   (AVNRT)**:

- A type of supraventricular tachycardia caused by a reentrant circuit within or around the AV node.
- It results in a rapid heart rate and can cause symptoms like palpitations, dizziness, and shortness of breath.

Herbs, Vitamins, Minerals, and Supplements for Supporting AV Node Function

Supporting the health and function of the AV node is essential for maintaining proper heart rhythm and preventing arrhythmias. Several herbs, vitamins, minerals, and supplements can help in this regard.

Herbs

1. **Hawthorn (Crataegus spp.):**
   - **Benefits**: Supports overall heart health and improves blood flow.
   - **Usage**: Available as tea, tincture, or in capsule form.
2. **Valerian Root (Valeriana officinalis):**

- **Benefits**: Calms the nervous
      system and helps regulate heart
      rate.
    - **Usage**: Available as tea, tincture,
      or in capsule form.
3. **Olive Leaf Extract (Olea
   europaea)**:
    - **Benefits**: Has antioxidant
      properties and supports
      cardiovascular health.
    - **Usage**: Available as capsules or
      liquid extract.
4. **Bilberry (Vaccinium myrtillus)**:
    - **Benefits**: Supports blood vessel
      health and improves circulation.
    - **Usage**: Available as tea, tincture,
      or in capsule form.

Vitamins

1. **Vitamin B6 (Pyridoxine)**:
    - **Benefits**: Supports nerve
      function and cardiovascular
      health.
    - **Sources**: Poultry, fish, potatoes,
      chickpeas.
    - **Supplementation**: Available in
      tablets or capsules.
2. **Vitamin B12 (Cobalamin)**:

- **Benefits**: Essential for nerve health and proper red blood cell formation.
    - **Sources**: Meat, dairy products, fortified cereals.
    - **Supplementation**: Available in tablets, capsules, or as injections.
3. **Folic Acid (Vitamin B9)**:
    - **Benefits**: Supports cardiovascular health by reducing homocysteine levels.
    - **Sources**: Leafy green vegetables, citrus fruits, beans.
    - **Supplementation**: Available in tablets or capsules.

Minerals

1. **Selenium**:
    - **Benefits**: Acts as an antioxidant and supports heart health.
    - **Sources**: Brazil nuts, seafood, meat.
    - **Supplementation**: Available in tablets or capsules.
2. **Zinc**:
    - **Benefits**: Supports immune function and cell growth.
    - **Sources**: Meat, shellfish, legumes.

- o **Supplementation**: Available in tablets or capsules.

3. **Iodine**:
   - o **Benefits**: Essential for thyroid function, which indirectly supports heart health.
   - o **Sources**: Iodized salt, seafood, dairy products.
   - o **Supplementation**: Available in tablets or as part of a multivitamin.

Supplements

1. **Resveratrol**:
   - o **Benefits**: Supports cardiovascular health and has antioxidant properties.
   - o **Sources**: Found in red wine, grapes, and berries.
   - o **Supplementation**: Available in capsule or liquid form.
2. **L-Arginine**:
   - o **Benefits**: An amino acid that supports nitric oxide production and improves blood flow.
   - o **Sources**: Meat, dairy, nuts, and seeds.
   - o **Supplementation**: Available in powder or capsule form.

3. **Astaxanthin**:
    - **Benefits**: A powerful antioxidant that supports cardiovascular health.
    - **Sources**: Found in algae, salmon, and other seafood.
    - **Supplementation**: Available in capsule form.
4. **Quercetin**:
    - **Benefits**: Supports cardiovascular health and has anti-inflammatory properties.
    - **Sources**: Found in apples, onions, and berries.
    - **Supplementation**: Available in tablet or capsule form

Arteries

Arteries are blood vessels that carry oxygenated blood away from the heart to various parts of the body. They are a crucial component of the cardiovascular system, ensuring that tissues receive the necessary oxygen and nutrients to function effectively.

Structure of Arteries

1. **Layers of Arterial Walls**:
   - **Tunica Intima**:
     - The innermost layer, consisting of a thin layer of endothelial cells that provide a smooth lining for blood to flow over.
     - Supported by a basement membrane and a layer of elastic fibers (internal elastic lamina).
   - **Tunica Media**:
     - The middle layer, composed mainly of smooth muscle cells and elastic fibers.
     - Responsible for regulating the diameter of the artery through contraction and

relaxation, thereby controlling blood pressure and flow.
- **Tunica Externa (Adventitia)**:
    - The outermost layer, composed of connective tissue that provides structural support and elasticity.
    - Contains nerves and smaller blood vessels (vasa vasorum) that supply the walls of larger arteries.

2. **Types of Arteries**:
    - **Elastic Arteries**:
        - Large arteries like the aorta and its major branches.
        - Contain a high proportion of elastic fibers in the tunica media, allowing them to stretch and recoil with each heartbeat.
    - **Muscular Arteries**:
        - Medium-sized arteries that distribute blood to specific organs and tissues.
        - Have a thicker tunica media with more smooth

muscle cells, allowing for
precise regulation of blood
flow through
vasoconstriction and
vasodilation.

- **Arterioles**:
  - The smallest type of
    arteries, leading into
    capillary networks.
  - Have a thin tunica media,
    which allows them to
    control blood flow into
    capillaries by constricting
    or dilating.

Function of Arteries

1. **Transportation of Oxygenated Blood**:
   - Arteries carry oxygen-rich blood
     from the heart to tissues
     throughout the body.
   - The only exception is the
     pulmonary arteries, which carry
     deoxygenated blood from the
     heart to the lungs for
     oxygenation.
2. **Regulation of Blood Pressure**:
   - Arterial walls, especially in
     muscular arteries and arterioles,

can constrict or dilate to regulate blood pressure and flow.

- This regulation ensures that blood reaches tissues under varying conditions, such as during exercise or rest.

3. **Pulsatile Flow**:
   - The elastic properties of large arteries allow them to absorb the pressure wave generated by the heart's contractions and maintain a steady flow of blood.

Arterial Health and Disease

1. **Atherosclerosis**:
   - A condition characterized by the buildup of plaques (composed of fats, cholesterol, and other substances) inside the arterial walls.
   - Can lead to narrowed and hardened arteries, reducing blood flow and increasing the risk of heart attack and stroke.
2. **Arterial Hypertension**:
   - Chronic high blood pressure can damage arterial walls, leading to conditions like atherosclerosis, aneurysms, and heart disease.

3. **Aneurysms**:
    - Abnormal bulges or weaknesses in the arterial wall, often caused by high blood pressure or atherosclerosis.
    - Can rupture, leading to life-threatening internal bleeding.

Herbs, Vitamins, Minerals, and Supplements for Arterial Health

Supporting arterial health is essential for maintaining overall cardiovascular health and preventing diseases like atherosclerosis and hypertension. Various herbs, vitamins, minerals, and supplements can help support and protect arterial health.

Herbs

1. **Garlic (Allium sativum)**:
    - **Benefits**: Reduces blood pressure, lowers cholesterol levels, and has anti-inflammatory properties.
    - **Usage**: Available as fresh garlic, capsules, or extracts.
2. **Ginkgo Biloba**:

- **Benefits**: Improves blood circulation and has antioxidant properties.
  - **Usage**: Available as capsules, tablets, or liquid extracts.
3. **Turmeric (Curcuma longa)**:
   - **Benefits**: Contains curcumin, which has anti-inflammatory and antioxidant effects.
   - **Usage**: Available as powder, capsules, or extracts.
4. **Hibiscus (Hibiscus sabdariffa)**:
   - **Benefits**: Lowers blood pressure and has antioxidant properties.
   - **Usage**: Available as tea, capsules, or extracts.

Vitamins

1. **Vitamin C (Ascorbic Acid)**:
   - **Benefits**: Supports collagen production for healthy arterial walls and acts as an antioxidant.
   - **Sources**: Citrus fruits, strawberries, bell peppers.
   - **Supplementation**: Available in tablets, capsules, or powder form.
2. **Vitamin E**:

- **Benefits**: Prevents oxidation of LDL cholesterol, which contributes to atherosclerosis.
  - **Sources**: Nuts, seeds, spinach, broccoli.
  - **Supplementation**: Available in capsules or tablets.

3. **Vitamin K2**:
  - **Benefits**: Helps direct calcium into bones and away from arteries, preventing calcification.
  - **Sources**: Fermented foods, cheese, egg yolks.
  - **Supplementation**: Available in capsules or tablets.

Minerals

1. **Magnesium**:
  - **Benefits**: Relaxes blood vessels, supports healthy blood pressure, and prevents arterial stiffness.
  - **Sources**: Green leafy vegetables, nuts, seeds.
  - **Supplementation**: Available in tablets, capsules, or as a powder.

2. **Potassium**:
  - **Benefits**: Helps regulate blood pressure by balancing sodium levels in the body.

o **Sources**: Bananas, oranges, potatoes, spinach.
   o **Supplementation**: Available in tablets or capsules.
3. **Calcium**:
   o **Benefits**: Necessary for vascular contraction and relaxation.
   o **Sources**: Dairy products, leafy green vegetables.
   o **Supplementation**: Available in tablets, capsules, or as a powder.

Supplements

1. **Omega-3 Fatty Acids**:
   o **Benefits**: Reduce inflammation, lower triglyceride levels, and support overall heart health.
   o **Sources**: Fatty fish, flaxseeds, walnuts.
   o **Supplementation**: Available in fish oil or flaxseed oil capsules.
2. **Coenzyme Q10 (CoQ10)**:
   o **Benefits**: Supports cellular energy production and has antioxidant properties.
   o **Sources**: Found in small amounts in meat and fish.
   o **Supplementation**: Available in capsule or softgel form.

3. **L-Arginine**:
   - **Benefits**: An amino acid that helps produce nitric oxide, which relaxes blood vessels and improves blood flow.
   - **Sources**: Meat, dairy, nuts, and seeds.
   - **Supplementation**: Available in powder or capsule form.
4. **Resveratrol**:
   - **Benefits**: Supports cardiovascular health and has antioxidant properties.
   - **Sources**: Found in red wine, grapes, and berries.
   - **Supplementation**: Available in capsule or liquid form.

Veins

Veins are blood vessels that carry deoxygenated blood from various parts of the body back to the heart. They play a crucial role in the circulatory system by ensuring that blood is returned for reoxygenation and nutrient replenishment.

Structure of Veins

1. **Layers of Venous Walls**:
    - **Tunica Intima**:
        - The innermost layer, composed of endothelial cells that provide a smooth surface for blood flow.
        - Contains valves that prevent the backflow of blood.
    - **Tunica Media**:
        - The middle layer, consisting of smooth muscle cells and elastic fibers, though it is thinner than that in arteries.
        - Less muscular and more flexible, allowing veins to accommodate varying volumes of blood.

- **Tunica Externa (Adventitia)**:
  - The outermost layer, made of connective tissue that provides structural support and elasticity.
  - Contains nerves and smaller blood vessels (vasa vasorum) that supply the walls of larger veins.

2. **Types of Veins**:
   - **Superficial Veins**:
     - Located close to the surface of the skin.
     - Often visible and are used for procedures like intravenous access or blood sampling.
   - **Deep Veins**:
     - Located deeper within the body, surrounded by muscle tissue.
     - Carry the majority of blood back to the heart and are often accompanied by corresponding arteries.
   - **Pulmonary Veins**:
     - Carry oxygenated blood from the lungs to the left atrium of the heart.

- ○ **Systemic Veins**:
    - ■ Carry deoxygenated blood from the rest of the body back to the right atrium of the heart.

Function of Veins

1. **Transportation of Deoxygenated Blood**:
   - ○ Veins carry deoxygenated blood from tissues back to the heart, except for the pulmonary veins, which carry oxygenated blood from the lungs.
2. **Volume Reservoir**:
   - ○ Veins can store large volumes of blood, acting as a reservoir. They can accommodate changes in blood volume by expanding or contracting.
3. **One-Way Valves**:
   - ○ Veins, particularly in the limbs, contain one-way valves that prevent the backflow of blood, ensuring it moves in one direction towards the heart.
4. **Venous Return Mechanisms**:
   - ○ **Skeletal Muscle Pump**: Muscle contractions compress

veins, pushing blood towards the heart.

- **Respiratory Pump**: During inhalation, pressure changes in the thoracic and abdominal cavities help move blood towards the heart.
- **Venomotor Tone**: The smooth muscle in the venous walls can contract to help push blood back to the heart.

Venous Health and Disease

1. **Varicose Veins**:
   - Enlarged and twisted veins, usually occurring in the legs due to valve failure, causing blood to pool.
   - Can cause pain, swelling, and skin changes.
2. **Chronic Venous Insufficiency (CVI)**:
   - A condition where veins have difficulty sending blood from the limbs back to the heart.
   - Can lead to symptoms like swelling, pain, and skin ulcers.
3. **Deep Vein Thrombosis (DVT)**:

- The formation of a blood clot in a deep vein, typically in the legs.
    - Can be life-threatening if the clot dislodges and travels to the lungs (pulmonary embolism).
4. **Phlebitis**:
    - Inflammation of a vein, often associated with blood clots (thrombophlebitis).
    - Can cause pain, swelling, and redness along the vein.

Herbs, Vitamins, Minerals, and Supplements for Venous Health

Supporting venous health is crucial for preventing conditions like varicose veins, CVI, and DVT. Various herbs, vitamins, minerals, and supplements can help support and protect venous function.

Herbs

1. **Horse Chestnut (Aesculus hippocastanum)**:
    - **Benefits**: Reduces symptoms of chronic venous insufficiency, such as swelling and pain.

- o **Usage**: Available as capsules, extracts, or topical creams.

2. **Butcher's Broom (Ruscus aculeatus):**
   - o **Benefits**: Supports vein tone and reduces swelling and inflammation.
   - o **Usage**: Available as capsules, extracts, or topical creams.

3. **Gotu Kola (Centella asiatica):**
   - o **Benefits**: Strengthens blood vessels, improves circulation, and reduces swelling.
   - o **Usage**: Available as capsules, extracts, or teas.

4. **Grape Seed Extract (Vitis vinifera):**
   - o **Benefits**: Contains antioxidants that support blood vessel health and reduce swelling.
   - o **Usage**: Available as capsules or extracts.

Vitamins

1. **Vitamin C (Ascorbic Acid):**
   - o **Benefits**: Supports collagen production for healthy vein walls and acts as an antioxidant.

- ○ **Sources**: Citrus fruits, strawberries, bell peppers.
- ○ **Supplementation**: Available in tablets, capsules, or powder form.

2. **Vitamin E:**
- ○ **Benefits**: Prevents oxidation of lipids and supports overall vascular health.
- ○ **Sources**: Nuts, seeds, spinach, broccoli.
- ○ **Supplementation**: Available in capsules or tablets.

3. **Vitamin K:**
- ○ **Benefits**: Essential for blood clotting and maintaining vein health.
- ○ **Sources**: Leafy green vegetables, broccoli, Brussels sprouts.
- ○ **Supplementation**: Available in tablets or capsules.

Minerals

1. **Magnesium:**
- ○ **Benefits**: Supports vascular health by relaxing blood vessels and improving blood flow.
- ○ **Sources**: Green leafy vegetables, nuts, seeds.

- **Supplementation**: Available in tablets, capsules, or as a powder.

2. **Copper**:
   - **Benefits**: Necessary for the formation of hemoglobin and maintaining the health of blood vessels.
   - **Sources**: Shellfish, nuts, seeds, whole grains.
   - **Supplementation**: Available in tablets or capsules.

3. **Zinc**:
   - **Benefits**: Supports immune function and wound healing, which is important for venous ulcers.
   - **Sources**: Meat, shellfish, legumes.
   - **Supplementation**: Available in tablets or capsules.

Supplements

1. **Diosmin**:
   - **Benefits**: Supports venous tone and reduces symptoms of venous insufficiency.
   - **Sources**: Found in citrus fruits.
   - **Supplementation**: Available in capsule or tablet form.

2. **Rutin**:
    - ○ **Benefits**: Strengthens blood vessels and reduces inflammation.
    - ○ **Sources**: Found in apples, citrus fruits, and buckwheat.
    - ○ **Supplementation**: Available in tablet or capsule form.
3. **Pycnogenol (Pine Bark Extract)**:
    - ○ **Benefits**: Contains antioxidants that support vascular health and reduce swelling.
    - ○ **Sources**: Derived from the bark of the French maritime pine tree.
    - ○ **Supplementation**: Available in capsules or tablets.
4. **Horse Chestnut Seed Extract**:
    - ○ **Benefits**: Reduces symptoms of venous insufficiency and supports vein health.
    - ○ **Sources**: Derived from the seeds of the horse chestnut tree.
    - ○ **Supplementation**: Available in capsules or topical creams.

Capillaries

Capillaries are the smallest blood vessels in the body, forming a network that connects arterioles to venules. They play a critical role in the exchange of oxygen, nutrients, and waste products between the blood and tissues.

Structure of Capillaries

1. **Layers of Capillary Walls**:
   - **Endothelial Layer**:
     - The single layer of endothelial cells forms the entire wall of a capillary.
     - These cells are thin and flat, allowing for easy diffusion of substances between the blood and surrounding tissues.
   - **Basement Membrane**:
     - A thin, extracellular matrix layer that supports the endothelial cells.
     - Provides structural integrity and regulates permeability.
2. **Types of Capillaries**:
   - **Continuous Capillaries**:

- The most common type, found in muscles, skin, lungs, and the central nervous system.
- Endothelial cells are closely joined, with small intercellular clefts that allow for selective permeability.
  - **Fenestrated Capillaries**:
    - Found in tissues with high rates of exchange, such as the kidneys, intestines, and endocrine glands.
    - Endothelial cells have pores (fenestrations) that increase permeability.
  - **Sinusoidal Capillaries**:
    - Found in the liver, spleen, and bone marrow.
    - Have larger gaps between endothelial cells, allowing the passage of larger molecules and cells.

Function of Capillaries

1. **Exchange of Gases**:
   - Oxygen from the blood diffuses through capillary walls into

tissues, while carbon dioxide from tissues diffuses into the blood to be carried away.

2. **Exchange of Nutrients and Waste Products**:
   - Nutrients such as glucose, amino acids, and fatty acids pass from the blood into tissues.
   - Waste products like urea and lactic acid diffuse from tissues into the blood for removal.

3. **Regulation of Blood Flow**:
   - Precapillary sphincters, rings of smooth muscle at the entrance to capillary beds, regulate blood flow into capillaries based on tissue needs.

4. **Fluid Exchange**:
   - Capillaries help maintain fluid balance by allowing the exchange of water and small solutes between blood plasma and interstitial fluid.

Capillary Health and Disease

1. **Capillary Fragility**:
   - Weak capillaries can lead to easy bruising and bleeding.

- Conditions like scurvy (vitamin C deficiency) can weaken capillary walls.
2. **Microangiopathy**:
   - A disease of the small blood vessels, including capillaries, often associated with diabetes.
   - Can lead to complications like diabetic retinopathy and nephropathy.
3. **Edema**:
   - Excess fluid accumulation in tissues due to increased capillary permeability or decreased lymphatic drainage.

Herbs, Vitamins, Minerals, and Supplements for Capillary Health

Supporting capillary health is essential for maintaining efficient nutrient and waste exchange and preventing capillary-related diseases. Various herbs, vitamins, minerals, and supplements can help support and protect capillary function.

Herbs

1. **Bilberry (Vaccinium myrtillus)**:
   - **Benefits**: Strengthens capillary walls, reduces permeability, and improves circulation.
   - **Usage**: Available as capsules, extracts, or dried berries.
2. **Horse Chestnut (Aesculus hippocastanum)**:
   - **Benefits**: Reduces capillary permeability and strengthens blood vessels.
   - **Usage**: Available as capsules, extracts, or topical creams.
3. **Ginkgo Biloba**:
   - **Benefits**: Improves blood flow and has antioxidant properties that protect capillaries.
   - **Usage**: Available as capsules, tablets, or liquid extracts.
4. **Gotu Kola (Centella asiatica)**:
   - **Benefits**: Strengthens blood vessels and improves circulation.
   - **Usage**: Available as capsules, extracts, or teas.

Vitamins

1. **Vitamin C (Ascorbic Acid):**
   - **Benefits**: Essential for collagen production, which maintains capillary strength and integrity.
   - **Sources**: Citrus fruits, strawberries, bell peppers.
   - **Supplementation**: Available in tablets, capsules, or powder form.
2. **Vitamin E:**
   - **Benefits**: Acts as an antioxidant, protecting capillaries from damage by free radicals.
   - **Sources**: Nuts, seeds, spinach, broccoli.
   - **Supplementation**: Available in capsules or tablets.
3. **Vitamin K:**
   - **Benefits**: Necessary for blood clotting and maintaining capillary health.
   - **Sources**: Leafy green vegetables, broccoli, Brussels sprouts.
   - **Supplementation**: Available in tablets or capsules.

Minerals

1. **Copper**:
   - **Benefits**: Essential for the formation of hemoglobin and maintaining the health of blood vessels.
   - **Sources**: Shellfish, nuts, seeds, whole grains.
   - **Supplementation**: Available in tablets or capsules.

2. **Zinc**:
   - **Benefits**: Supports immune function and wound healing, important for maintaining healthy capillaries.
   - **Sources**: Meat, shellfish, legumes.
   - **Supplementation**: Available in tablets or capsules.

3. **Manganese**:
   - **Benefits**: Involved in the formation of connective tissue, including capillary walls.
   - **Sources**: Nuts, seeds, whole grains.
   - **Supplementation**: Available in tablets or capsules.

1. **Rutin**:
    - ○ **Benefits**: Strengthens blood vessels and reduces capillary fragility.
    - ○ **Sources**: Found in apples, citrus fruits, and buckwheat.
    - ○ **Supplementation**: Available in tablet or capsule form.
2. **Pycnogenol (Pine Bark Extract)**:
    - ○ **Benefits**: Contains antioxidants that support capillary health and reduce permeability.
    - ○ **Sources**: Derived from the bark of the French maritime pine tree.
    - ○ **Supplementation**: Available in capsules or tablets.
3. **Diosmin**:
    - ○ **Benefits**: Supports venous tone and reduces capillary permeability.
    - ○ **Sources**: Found in citrus fruits.
    - ○ **Supplementation**: Available in capsule or tablet form.
4. **Bioflavonoids**:
    - ○ **Benefits**: Enhance the effects of vitamin C and improve capillary strength and permeability.

- o **Sources**: Citrus fruits, berries, green tea.
- o **Supplementation**: Available in capsules or tablets.

Red Blood Cells (Erythrocytes)

Red blood cells (RBCs), or erythrocytes, are essential components of the blood, primarily responsible for transporting oxygen from the lungs to the tissues and carbon dioxide from the tissues back to the lungs.

Structure of Red Blood Cells

1. **Shape and Size**:
   - **Biconcave Disc Shape**: This shape increases the surface area-to-volume ratio, facilitating efficient gas exchange.
   - **Diameter**: Typically about 6-8 micrometers.
   - **Thickness**: Approximately 2 micrometers at the thickest point and 1 micrometer at the center.
2. **Composition**:
   - **Hemoglobin**: The protein that binds to oxygen. Each RBC contains approximately 270 million hemoglobin molecules.
   - **Cell Membrane**: A flexible lipid bilayer with embedded proteins that provide structural integrity and flexibility, allowing RBCs to traverse narrow capillaries.

- ○ **No Nucleus**: Mature RBCs lack a nucleus and most organelles, maximizing space for hemoglobin.

Function of Red Blood Cells

1. **Oxygen Transport**:
   - ○ **Binding in the Lungs**: RBCs pick up oxygen in the alveoli of the lungs, where oxygen concentration is high.
   - ○ **Release in Tissues**: Oxygen is released in tissues where it is needed, facilitated by the lower oxygen concentration and the presence of carbon dioxide.
2. **Carbon Dioxide Transport**:
   - ○ **From Tissues to Lungs**: Carbon dioxide, a waste product of cellular respiration, is transported back to the lungs in three forms:
     - Dissolved in plasma.
     - Chemically bound to hemoglobin (forming carbaminohemoglobin).
     - As bicarbonate ions (HCO_3^-) formed in RBCs and transported in plasma.

3. **Buffering Blood pH**:
    - **Hemoglobin Buffering**:
      Hemoglobin helps to buffer blood
      pH by binding to excess hydrogen
      ions (H^+), preventing significant
      changes in pH.

Production and Lifespan

1. **Erythropoiesis (Production)**:
    - **Location**: Occurs in the red
      bone marrow of long bones, ribs,
      sternum, and pelvis.
    - **Process**: Hematopoietic stem
      cells differentiate into
      proerythroblasts, which further
      mature into erythroblasts and
      then reticulocytes before
      becoming mature erythrocytes.
    - **Regulation**: Controlled by
      erythropoietin (EPO), a hormone
      produced by the kidneys in
      response to low oxygen levels.
2. **Lifespan and Destruction**:
    - **Lifespan**: Approximately 120
      days.
    - **Destruction**: Old or damaged
      RBCs are phagocytosed by
      macrophages in the spleen, liver,
      and bone marrow. Hemoglobin is

broken down, and its components are recycled.

Disorders Related to Red Blood Cells

1. **Anemia**:
   - **Iron-Deficiency Anemia**: Caused by insufficient iron, leading to reduced hemoglobin production.
   - **Pernicious Anemia**: Caused by vitamin B12 deficiency due to impaired absorption.
   - **Hemolytic Anemia**: Caused by the premature destruction of RBCs.
   - **Sickle Cell Anemia**: A genetic disorder leading to the production of abnormal hemoglobin, causing RBCs to become rigid and sickle-shaped.
2. **Polycythemia**:
   - **Polycythemia Vera**: A bone marrow disorder leading to excessive RBC production.
   - **Secondary Polycythemia**: Caused by increased EPO production due to chronic hypoxia (e.g., high altitude, chronic lung disease).

Herbs, Vitamins, Minerals, and Supplements for Red Blood Cells

Supporting red blood cell health is crucial for maintaining adequate oxygen transport and overall well-being. Various nutrients and supplements can aid in the formation, maintenance, and health of RBCs.

Herbs

1. **Nettle (Urtica dioica):**
    - **Benefits**: Rich in iron and vitamin C, supports overall blood health and hemoglobin production.
    - **Usage**: Can be consumed as a tea, tincture, or capsule.
2. **Dandelion (Taraxacum officinale):**
    - **Benefits**: Contains vitamins and minerals that support RBC health.
    - **Usage**: Commonly used in teas, extracts, or salads.
3. **Yellow Dock (Rumex crispus):**
    - **Benefits**: High in iron and helps in the detoxification process,

supporting liver health and blood purification.

- o **Usage**: Available as tinctures, capsules, or teas.

Vitamins

1. **Vitamin B12 (Cobalamin)**:
   - o **Benefits**: Essential for DNA synthesis and the proper formation of RBCs.
   - o **Sources**: Found in animal products such as meat, fish, dairy, and eggs.
   - o **Supplementation**: Available in tablets, capsules, or injections.
2. **Folic Acid (Vitamin B9)**:
   - o **Benefits**: Necessary for DNA synthesis and RBC production.
   - o **Sources**: Leafy greens, legumes, nuts, and fortified cereals.
   - o **Supplementation**: Available in tablets or capsules.
3. **Vitamin C (Ascorbic Acid)**:
   - o **Benefits**: Enhances iron absorption from plant-based sources and supports overall immune function.
   - o **Sources**: Citrus fruits, berries, bell peppers, and leafy greens.

- ○ **Supplementation**: Available in tablets, capsules, or powders.

Minerals

1. **Iron:**
   - ○ **Benefits**: Crucial for hemoglobin production and oxygen transport.
   - ○ **Sources**: Red meat, poultry, fish, beans, lentils, and fortified cereals.
   - ○ **Supplementation**: Available in tablets, capsules, or liquid form.
2. **Copper:**
   - ○ **Benefits**: Aids in iron absorption and the formation of hemoglobin.
   - ○ **Sources**: Shellfish, nuts, seeds, and whole grains.
   - ○ **Supplementation**: Available in tablets or capsules.
3. **Zinc:**
   - ○ **Benefits**: Supports immune function and overall health, indirectly supporting RBC production.
   - ○ **Sources**: Meat, shellfish, legumes, seeds, and nuts.
   - ○ **Supplementation**: Available in tablets or capsules.

Supplements

1. **Iron Supplements**:
   - **Benefits**: Used to treat iron-deficiency anemia and support healthy RBC levels.
   - **Forms**: Ferrous sulfate, ferrous gluconate, ferrous fumarate.
2. **Vitamin B12 Supplements**:
   - **Benefits**: Used to treat B12 deficiency and support RBC production.
   - **Forms**: Cyanocobalamin, methylcobalamin.
3. **Folic Acid Supplements**:
   - **Benefits**: Used to prevent and treat folate deficiency anemia.
   - **Forms**: Available in tablets or capsules.
4. **Spirulina**:
   - **Benefits**: A blue-green algae rich in vitamins, minerals, and proteins, supporting overall blood health.
   - **Usage**: Available in powder, tablet, or capsule form.

Red blood cells are vital for oxygen transport and overall health. Understanding their structure, function, and the nutrients that support their health can help maintain optimal RBC function and prevent related disorders.

Incorporating specific herbs, vitamins, minerals, and supplements into your diet can support RBC health and enhance overall well-being. Always consult with a healthcare provider before starting any new supplement regimen, especially if you have existing health conditions or are taking medications.

White Blood Cells (Leukocytes)

White blood cells (WBCs), or leukocytes, are crucial components of the immune system, responsible for defending the body against infections, foreign invaders, and diseases. They are produced in the bone marrow and circulate in the blood and lymphatic system.

Types of White Blood Cells

1. **Granulocytes**:
   - **Neutrophils**:
     - Most abundant type of WBC.
     - Primary role in fighting bacterial infections.
     - Contain granules with enzymes that digest microorganisms.
   - **Eosinophils**:
     - Combat parasitic infections and are involved in allergic reactions.
     - Contain granules with toxic proteins and enzymes.
   - **Basophils**:
     - Least common type of WBC.

- Release histamine during allergic reactions and help combat parasites.

2. **Agranulocytes**:
    - **Lymphocytes**:
        - B cells: Produce antibodies to neutralize pathogens.
        - T cells: Destroy infected or cancerous cells and coordinate the immune response.
        - Natural Killer (NK) cells: Attack and destroy tumor cells and virally infected cells.
    - **Monocytes**:
        - Differentiate into macrophages and dendritic cells in tissues.
        - Phagocytize pathogens and dead cells and present antigens to T cells.

Structure of White Blood Cells

1. **Nucleus**:
    - Prominent and varies in shape among different types of WBCs.

- Multilobed in granulocytes; large and round in lymphocytes; kidney-shaped in monocytes.

2. **Cytoplasm**:
   - Contains granules in granulocytes that store enzymes and other chemicals.
   - Agranulocytes have clear cytoplasm without visible granules under a light microscope.

Function of White Blood Cells

1. **Phagocytosis**:
   - Neutrophils and monocytes (as macrophages) engulf and digest pathogens and debris.
2. **Antibody Production**:
   - B cells produce antibodies that specifically target and neutralize pathogens.
3. **Cell-Mediated Immunity**:
   - T cells attack and destroy infected or cancerous cells.
4. **Allergic Response**:
   - Eosinophils and basophils release substances like histamine that mediate allergic reactions.
5. **Immune Surveillance**:

- NK cells monitor and destroy abnormal cells in the body.

Production and Lifespan

1. **Production:**
   - Occurs in the bone marrow from hematopoietic stem cells.
   - Different growth factors and cytokines regulate the production of specific types of WBCs.
2. **Lifespan:**
   - Varies widely among different types.
   - Neutrophils: Few hours to days.
   - Lymphocytes: Can live from a few days to several years.
   - Monocytes: Circulate in blood for 1-3 days, then differentiate into macrophages in tissues where they can live for months.

Disorders Related to White Blood Cells

1. **Leukopenia:**
   - Low WBC count, increasing infection risk.
   - Can result from bone marrow disorders, autoimmune diseases,

severe infections, or certain
medications.

2. **Leukocytosis**:
   - High WBC count, often a
     response to infection or
     inflammation.
   - Can indicate stress,
     inflammation, leukemia, or other
     conditions.

3. **Leukemia**:
   - A group of cancers affecting the
     bone marrow and blood, leading
     to the overproduction of
     abnormal WBCs.
   - Types include acute
     lymphoblastic leukemia (ALL),
     chronic lymphocytic leukemia
     (CLL), acute myeloid leukemia
     (AML), and chronic myeloid
     leukemia (CML).

Herbs, Vitamins, Minerals, and Supplements for White Blood Cells

Supporting white blood cell health can enhance
the immune system's ability to fight infections
and maintain overall health. Various nutrients

and supplements can aid in the formation, maintenance, and function of WBCs.

Herbs

1. **Echinacea (Echinacea purpurea):**
   - **Benefits**: Boosts immune function by increasing WBC production and activity.
   - **Usage**: Available as teas, tinctures, or capsules.
2. **Astragalus (Astragalus membranaceus):**
   - **Benefits**: Enhances immune function and increases WBC count.
   - **Usage**: Commonly used in teas, soups, or as supplements.
3. **Garlic (Allium sativum):**
   - **Benefits**: Has antimicrobial properties and can stimulate immune function.
   - **Usage**: Can be consumed fresh, as a supplement, or in cooking.

Vitamins

1. **Vitamin C (Ascorbic Acid):**

- **Benefits**: Supports the immune system by enhancing WBC function and production.
- **Sources**: Citrus fruits, berries, bell peppers, and leafy greens.
- **Supplementation**: Available in tablets, capsules, or powders.

2. **Vitamin D**:
   - **Benefits**: Modulates the immune response and supports WBC function.
   - **Sources**: Sunlight exposure, fatty fish, fortified foods.
   - **Supplementation**: Available in tablets, capsules, or liquids.

3. **Vitamin E**:
   - **Benefits**: Acts as an antioxidant and supports WBC health.
   - **Sources**: Nuts, seeds, and vegetable oils.
   - **Supplementation**: Available in tablets, capsules, or softgels.

Minerals

1. **Zinc**:
   - **Benefits**: Essential for the development and function of immune cells.

- ○ **Sources**: Meat, shellfish, legumes, seeds, and nuts.
  - ○ **Supplementation**: Available in tablets, capsules, or lozenges.

2. **Selenium**:
   - ○ **Benefits**: Supports immune function and protects against oxidative stress.
   - ○ **Sources**: Brazil nuts, seafood, and meats.
   - ○ **Supplementation**: Available in tablets or capsules.

3. **Iron**:
   - ○ **Benefits**: Essential for the proliferation and maturation of WBCs.
   - ○ **Sources**: Red meat, poultry, fish, beans, lentils, and fortified cereals.
   - ○ **Supplementation**: Available in tablets, capsules, or liquid form.

Supplements

1. **Probiotics**:
   - ○ **Benefits**: Support gut health and enhance the immune response.
   - ○ **Forms**: Available in capsules, tablets, powders, or fermented foods like yogurt and kefir.

2. **Omega-3 Fatty Acids**:
   - ○ **Benefits**: Reduce inflammation and support immune function.
   - ○ **Sources**: Fatty fish, flaxseeds, chia seeds.
   - ○ **Supplementation**: Available in fish oil or flaxseed oil capsules.
3. **Colostrum**:
   - ○ **Benefits**: Rich in antibodies and immune-boosting compounds.
   - ○ **Sources**: Available as powders or capsules derived from bovine colostrum.

White blood cells are essential for immune defense, protecting the body against infections and diseases. Understanding their structure, function, and the nutrients that support their health can help maintain a robust immune system. Incorporating specific herbs, vitamins, minerals, and supplements into your diet can support WBC health and enhance overall immune function. Always consult with a healthcare provider before starting any new supplement regimen, especially if you have existing health conditions or are taking medications.

Platelets (Thrombocytes)

Platelets, or thrombocytes, are small, disc-shaped cell fragments in the blood that are essential for blood clotting and wound healing. They play a crucial role in hemostasis, the process that stops bleeding at the site of an injured blood vessel.

Structure of Platelets

1. **Size and Shape:**
   - Diameter: About 2-3 micrometers.
   - Shape: Small, irregularly shaped cell fragments without a nucleus.
2. **Components:**
   - **Membrane:** Contains receptors essential for platelet adhesion and aggregation.
   - **Granules:** Contain clotting factors, enzymes, and other proteins necessary for hemostasis. Granules are of two types:
     - **Alpha Granules:** Contain proteins such as fibrinogen, von Willebrand factor, and platelet-derived growth factor.

- **Dense Granules**: Contain ADP, ATP, calcium, and serotonin.

Function of Platelets

1. **Hemostasis**:
   - **Vascular Spasm**: Immediate constriction of the blood vessel to reduce blood flow.
   - **Platelet Plug Formation**: Platelets adhere to exposed collagen fibers at the injury site and aggregate to form a temporary plug.
   - **Coagulation**: Clotting factors in the blood plasma are activated in a cascade, resulting in the conversion of fibrinogen to fibrin, which stabilizes the platelet plug.
2. **Wound Healing**:
   - **Growth Factors**: Released from alpha granules to stimulate tissue repair and regeneration.
   - **Inflammation**: Platelets release signals that recruit immune cells to the site of injury.

Production and Lifespan

1. **Thrombopoiesis (Production)**:
    - **Location**: Occurs in the bone marrow.
    - **Process**: Megakaryocytes, large bone marrow cells, produce platelets by shedding cytoplasmic fragments.
    - **Regulation**: Controlled by thrombopoietin, a hormone produced primarily by the liver and kidneys.
2. **Lifespan**:
    - Approximately 7-10 days in circulation.
    - Old or damaged platelets are removed by the spleen and liver.

Disorders Related to Platelets

1. **Thrombocytopenia**:
    - **Low Platelet Count**: Increases the risk of bleeding.
    - **Causes**: Bone marrow disorders, autoimmune diseases, certain medications, and severe infections.
2. **Thrombocytosis**:
    - **High Platelet Count**: Increases the risk of thrombosis (blood clots).

- **Causes**: Bone marrow disorders, inflammation, and certain cancers.
3. **Platelet Dysfunction**:
   - **Impaired Function**: Can occur due to genetic disorders, medications (e.g., aspirin), or medical conditions.
   - **Effects**: Leads to abnormal bleeding despite a normal platelet count.

Herbs, Vitamins, Minerals, and Supplements for Platelet Health

Supporting platelet health is crucial for maintaining proper blood clotting and wound healing. Various nutrients and supplements can aid in the formation, maintenance, and function of platelets.

Herbs

1. **Ginger (Zingiber officinale)**:
   - **Benefits**: Contains compounds that support blood circulation and prevent excessive platelet aggregation.

- ○ **Usage**: Can be consumed as tea, fresh or dried in cooking, or as supplements.
2. **Ginkgo Biloba**:
   - ○ **Benefits**: Enhances blood flow and has anticoagulant properties, helping to maintain balanced platelet function.
   - ○ **Usage**: Available in capsules, tablets, or extracts.
3. **Turmeric (Curcuma longa)**:
   - ○ **Benefits**: Contains curcumin, which has anti-inflammatory and anticoagulant properties.
   - ○ **Usage**: Used in cooking, or as supplements in capsules or extracts.

Vitamins

1. **Vitamin K**:
   - ○ **Benefits**: Essential for the synthesis of clotting factors and proper platelet function.
   - ○ **Sources**: Leafy green vegetables, broccoli, Brussels sprouts, and fermented foods.
   - ○ **Supplementation**: Available in tablets, capsules, or liquid form.
2. **Vitamin B12 (Cobalamin)**:

- o **Benefits**: Necessary for the production of healthy blood cells, including platelets.
    - o **Sources**: Meat, fish, dairy, and fortified cereals.
    - o **Supplementation**: Available in tablets, capsules, or injections.
3. **Vitamin C (Ascorbic Acid)**:
    - o **Benefits**: Supports overall immune function and helps maintain the integrity of blood vessels.
    - o **Sources**: Citrus fruits, berries, bell peppers, and leafy greens.
    - o **Supplementation**: Available in tablets, capsules, or powders.

Minerals

1. **Iron**:
    - o **Benefits**: Essential for the production of hemoglobin and healthy blood cells.
    - o **Sources**: Red meat, poultry, fish, beans, lentils, and fortified cereals.
    - o **Supplementation**: Available in tablets, capsules, or liquid form.
2. **Magnesium**:

- o **Benefits**: Plays a role in blood clotting and maintaining healthy blood vessels.
  - o **Sources**: Nuts, seeds, whole grains, and leafy green vegetables.
  - o **Supplementation**: Available in tablets, capsules, or powders.

3. **Zinc**:
   - o **Benefits**: Supports immune function and wound healing, indirectly supporting platelet function.
   - o **Sources**: Meat, shellfish, legumes, seeds, and nuts.
   - o **Supplementation**: Available in tablets or capsules.

Supplements

1. **Omega-3 Fatty Acids**:
   - o **Benefits**: Have anti-inflammatory properties and help maintain balanced platelet function.
   - o **Sources**: Fatty fish, flaxseeds, chia seeds.
   - o **Supplementation**: Available in fish oil or flaxseed oil capsules.
2. **Bromelain**:

- Benefits: An enzyme found in pineapples that has anti-inflammatory and anticoagulant properties.
  - **Usage**: Available as a supplement in tablet or capsule form.
3. **Coenzyme Q10 (CoQ10):**
   - **Benefits**: Supports overall cardiovascular health and energy production in cells.
   - **Usage**: Available in tablets, capsules, or softgels.

Platelets are vital for blood clotting and wound healing. Understanding their structure, function, and the nutrients that support their health can help maintain proper platelet function and prevent related disorders. Incorporating specific herbs, vitamins, minerals, and supplements into your diet can support platelet health and enhance overall well-being. Always consult with a healthcare provider before starting any new supplement regimen, especially if you have existing health conditions or are taking medications.

Plasma

Plasma is the liquid component of blood, comprising about 55% of its total volume. It serves as the medium for transporting nutrients, hormones, waste products, and other substances throughout the body. Plasma is essential for maintaining blood pressure and volume and plays a crucial role in immune function and blood clotting.

Composition of Plasma

1. **Water:**
   - Makes up about 90-92% of plasma.
   - Functions as a solvent and helps in the transportation of substances.
2. **Proteins:**
   - **Albumin**: The most abundant plasma protein, responsible for maintaining osmotic pressure and transporting hormones, drugs, and other substances.
   - **Globulins**: Includes antibodies (immunoglobulins) that are essential for immune response.
   - **Fibrinogen**: A key protein in blood clotting.

o **Regulatory Proteins**:
   Hormones and enzymes that
   regulate various physiological
   processes.

3. **Electrolytes**:
   o Includes sodium, potassium,
     calcium, magnesium, chloride,
     bicarbonate, phosphate, and
     sulfate.
   o Maintains pH balance, osmotic
     pressure, and cellular function.

4. **Nutrients**:
   o Glucose, amino acids, lipids, and
     vitamins absorbed from the
     digestive tract and transported to
     cells for energy and growth.

5. **Waste Products**:
   o Includes urea, creatinine,
     bilirubin, and ammonia, which
     are transported to the kidneys,
     liver, and lungs for excretion.

6. **Gases**:
   o Oxygen and carbon dioxide
     transported between the lungs
     and tissues.

7. **Hormones**:
   o Chemical messengers that
     regulate various body functions.

Function of Plasma

1. **Transportation**:
    - Carries nutrients, hormones, and waste products to and from cells.
    - Transports blood cells throughout the body.
2. **Regulation**:
    - Maintains blood pressure and volume.
    - Helps regulate body temperature by distributing heat.
3. **Protection**:
    - Contains antibodies and proteins involved in immune response.
    - Contains clotting factors that prevent excessive bleeding.

Disorders Related to Plasma

1. **Hypovolemia**:
    - Low blood plasma volume, often due to dehydration or blood loss.
    - Symptoms: Weakness, dizziness, low blood pressure.
2. **Hypervolemia**:
    - High blood plasma volume, often due to kidney failure or heart failure.
    - Symptoms: Swelling, high blood pressure, shortness of breath.
3. **Plasma Protein Disorders**:

- Includes conditions like hypoalbuminemia (low albumin levels) and hyperglobulinemia (high globulin levels).
- Can be caused by liver disease, kidney disease, or chronic infections.

Herbs, Vitamins, Minerals, and Supplements for Plasma Health

Supporting plasma health is essential for overall well-being, as plasma plays a critical role in transporting nutrients, maintaining hydration, and supporting immune function.

Herbs

1. **Dandelion (Taraxacum officinale)**:
   - **Benefits**: Acts as a diuretic, helping to balance fluid levels and support liver function.
   - **Usage**: Can be consumed as tea, tincture, or in salads.
2. **Nettle (Urtica dioica)**:
   - **Benefits**: Rich in vitamins and minerals, supports detoxification and kidney function.
   - **Usage**: Available as tea, capsules, or tinctures.

3. **Milk Thistle (Silybum marianum):**
    - **Benefits**: Supports liver health, which is crucial for plasma protein production.
    - **Usage**: Available in capsules, tablets, or tinctures.

Vitamins

1. **Vitamin C (Ascorbic Acid):**
    - **Benefits**: Supports immune function and antioxidant defense.
    - **Sources**: Citrus fruits, berries, bell peppers, and leafy greens.
    - **Supplementation**: Available in tablets, capsules, or powders.
2. **Vitamin K:**
    - **Benefits**: Essential for blood clotting and maintaining normal plasma levels.
    - **Sources**: Leafy green vegetables, broccoli, Brussels sprouts, and fermented foods.
    - **Supplementation**: Available in tablets, capsules, or liquid form.
3. **B Vitamins (B6, B12, Folate):**
    - **Benefits**: Support red blood cell production and overall blood health.

- ○ **Sources**: Meat, fish, dairy, eggs, leafy greens, and fortified cereals.
- ○ **Supplementation**: Available in tablets, capsules, or injections.

Minerals

1. **Iron**:
   - ○ **Benefits**: Essential for hemoglobin production and oxygen transport.
   - ○ **Sources**: Red meat, poultry, fish, beans, lentils, and fortified cereals.
   - ○ **Supplementation**: Available in tablets, capsules, or liquid form.
2. **Magnesium**:
   - ○ **Benefits**: Supports muscle and nerve function, and helps maintain normal blood pressure.
   - ○ **Sources**: Nuts, seeds, whole grains, and leafy green vegetables.
   - ○ **Supplementation**: Available in tablets, capsules, or powders.
3. **Calcium**:
   - ○ **Benefits**: Essential for blood clotting and muscle function.
   - ○ **Sources**: Dairy products, leafy greens, and fortified foods.

- o **Supplementation**: Available in tablets, capsules, or chews.

Supplements

1. **Omega-3 Fatty Acids**:
   - o **Benefits**: Reduce inflammation and support cardiovascular health.
   - o **Sources**: Fatty fish, flaxseeds, chia seeds.
   - o **Supplementation**: Available in fish oil or flaxseed oil capsules.
2. **Probiotics**:
   - o **Benefits**: Support gut health, which is essential for nutrient absorption and overall plasma health.
   - o **Forms**: Available in capsules, tablets, powders, or fermented foods like yogurt and kefir.
3. **Coenzyme Q10 (CoQ10)**:
   - o **Benefits**: Supports cardiovascular health and energy production in cells.
   - o **Usage**: Available in tablets, capsules, or softgels.

Plasma is a vital component of blood, responsible for transporting nutrients, hormones, and waste products, maintaining hydration and blood pressure, and supporting immune function. Understanding its composition and functions helps in maintaining overall health. Incorporating specific herbs, vitamins, minerals, and supplements into your diet can support plasma health and enhance overall well-being. Always consult with a healthcare provider before starting any new supplement regimen, especially if you have existing health conditions or are taking medications.

Conclusion

In our exploration of the cardiovascular system, we've delved into the intricate network that sustains life by delivering oxygen and nutrients to every cell and removing waste products. From the beating heart, with its chambers and valves, to the vast web of arteries, veins, and capillaries, the cardiovascular system is a marvel of biological engineering. Understanding its components—the heart, blood vessels, and blood cells—illuminates the profound complexity and resilience of the human body.

Our journey through the cardiovascular system highlights the crucial role of maintaining its health for overall well-being. Embracing a holistic approach that incorporates herbs, vitamins, minerals, and supplements can offer natural support for cardiovascular function. Whether it's the heart-strengthening properties of hawthorn, the anti-inflammatory benefits of omega-3 fatty acids, or the blood-boosting power of iron, nature provides a rich pharmacy to nourish and protect our hearts.

Nature's bounty offers an array of remedies that can help prevent and manage cardiovascular conditions. Herbs like garlic and turmeric possess potent anti-inflammatory and antioxidant properties, while vitamins such as B6, B12, and folate play critical roles in reducing homocysteine levels, a risk factor for heart disease. Minerals like magnesium and potassium are essential for maintaining healthy blood pressure and cardiac rhythm, and supplements like CoQ10 support cellular energy production and heart health.

Incorporating these natural elements into your daily routine doesn't have to be complicated. Simple dietary adjustments, such as increasing your intake of leafy greens, nuts, seeds, and fatty fish, can make a significant difference. Herbal teas, tinctures, and supplements can further enhance your cardiovascular health regimen. However, it's important to approach these changes thoughtfully and consult with healthcare professionals to tailor a plan that meets your specific needs.

Beyond diet and supplements, lifestyle factors play a pivotal role in cardiovascular health. Regular physical activity, stress management, adequate sleep, and avoiding harmful habits like smoking are all essential. By embracing a heart-healthy lifestyle, you not only support your cardiovascular system but also enhance your overall quality of life.

The natural path to healing your cardiovascular system is not a quick fix but a lifelong journey. It involves making informed choices, staying committed to healthy habits, and being proactive about your heart health. By integrating the wisdom of natural remedies with modern medical advice, you can create a balanced and sustainable approach to cardiovascular wellness.

Your cardiovascular system is the lifeline of your body, deserving of care and attention. Through the synergistic power of natural remedies and a heart-healthy lifestyle, you can nurture your heart and vascular system, ensuring vitality and longevity. Let this journey be a testament to the remarkable potential of natural healing and the enduring strength of the human heart.

Legal Disclaimer

The information provided in "The Natural Path to Healing Your Cardiovascular System" is intended for general knowledge and educational purposes only. It is not a substitute for professional medical advice, diagnosis, or treatment. Always seek the advice of your physician or other qualified health providers with any questions you may have regarding a medical condition or before starting any new health regimen, including dietary changes, supplements, or exercise programs.

The authors and publishers of this book are not responsible for any adverse effects or consequences resulting from the use of any suggestions, preparations, or procedures described within this book. The use of any information provided in this book is solely at your own risk. If you have or suspect that you have a medical problem, promptly contact your healthcare provider.

The contents of this book are based on the research and opinions of the authors. The authors have made every effort to provide accurate and up-to-date information, but medical knowledge is constantly evolving, and thus the accuracy of the information contained herein cannot be guaranteed.

Consult with your healthcare provider before making any decisions related to your health, particularly if you are pregnant, nursing, have existing medical conditions, or are taking prescription medications.

The authors and publishers disclaim any liability for any loss, injury, or damage incurred as a consequence, directly or indirectly, of the use and application of any of the contents of this book.

Meet the Author

Hey everyone, just wanted to invite everyone to join me on my social pages. Links below!

Facebook Page....Luna Parnell's Written Works

Patreon page.... patreon.com/Lunastreasures